19 Dormant physiological Reserve

23 This is the new self-vision we must hold.

24 Heart Rate variability

26 very interesting brain connection 27 BIRDsong?

# SECRETS OF AGING WELL GET OUTSIDE

## THE FITNESS YOU CAN'T GET IN A GYM

Be Healthier, Recharge Your Brain, Prevent Burnout, Find More Joy, And Maybe Live To Be 100

MARTIN PAZZANI

# SECRETS OF AGING WELL GET OUTSIDE

## THE FITNESS YOU CAN'T GET IN A GYM

Be Healthier, Recharge Your Brain, Prevent Burnout, Find More Joy, And Maybe Live To Be 100

MARTIN PAZZANI

Niche Pressworks

Indianapolis

Get Outside

ISBN-13: 978-1-952654-08-4 eBook
978-1-952654-09-1 Paperback
978-1-952654-11-4 Hardback



Thank you to all my fellow hikers who were eager to share their stories and their photos. We received hundreds of contributions and distilled a nice collection of them in this book along with their personal snapshots. We've done our best to optimize the quality for this printed version. To see more stories and full color images...please visit our website. To share your own pictures and stories for Book Two, please go to www.getoutside.online/hikerstories.



Published by Niche Pressworks; http://NichePressworks.com

# DEDICATION

*To Mom and Dad*

# TABLE OF CONTENTS

# PREFACE

*I have sampled this life.*

—MARK TWAIN

As I write this, I'm 64.

I have mountains of experience—five million air miles and over 100,000,000 uphill steps spent hiking and climbing across seven continents. I've had a long career in business and marketing—in small companies, global mega-companies, and across many industries. Some might say I've been around.

It's taken over five decades to accumulate those miles, steps, and hills. I can't begin to tell you how many times I've stumbled and fallen flat on my face, chickened out and turned around, or walked many miles in the wrong direction. There have been lots of scrapes and bruises, some broken bones, and even a few near-death experiences. I've spent, lost, and passed up a lot of money on the road less traveled. But the experience and the lessons learned have been so worth it, because as they say, "No pain, no gain." I believe that wholeheartedly.

You see, I'm compulsively curious about the world, and I have always wanted to explore it. But, instead of the explorer-geologist-astronaut I dreamed of being as a teen, I somehow wound up in the corporate world. So, it was only natural that I found ways to explore anyway and, as a result, have sandwiched plenty of hiking and climbing into forty years of business experience. I was fortunate to be able to do climbing expeditions and treks to Antarctica and Nepal, across North and South America, the Alps, Africa, and countless climbs of Mount Washington in New Hampshire.

My business experience has been just as wide-ranging. First, there was a charge up the corporate ladder to senior management in global mega-corporations that had me working across six of those continents. Then serial entrepreneur in numerous startups (some worked, most did not). Madison Avenue advertising business. A term as the CEO of a music company. Went to a few TED Conferences and gave a TED Talk. And senior management of the world's largest fitness company.

My whirlwind of different business experiences, perspectives, and challenges bring a lot of variety to the table. An executive recruiter recently called me a "marketing Swiss army knife," which I kind of liked. As I said, I'm really grateful and fortunate to have had those experiences.

I've been immersed in the fitness business and in the world of outdoor adventure for a very long time—as a participant, a student, an executive, and an entrepreneur. My passion for fitness led me to found a think tank that studies the science behind longevity, brain health, and functional fitness with the intent of creating an "upstream preventive healthcare" company focused on the specific needs of people above age 45.

I've also observed that while we are indeed living longer, we have not figured out how to live with this new longevity. Many of us are too passive and inactive. We rely on outdated ideas about aging where medicine and drugs keep us alive, and surgery patches us up. We seem to be always looking for a magic pill that will be the fountain of youth.

But here's the secret. You won't find the fountain of youth in a doctor's office. Having worked with many top fitness trainers and some of the best high-altitude mountain climbers and guides in the world, I've benefited from their guidance. I've worked and lived in a wide range of places, industries, and roles. Along the way, I was lucky enough to have a never-ending variety of interesting colleagues, collaborators, mentors, detractors, critics, and competitors. I'm a sponge, and I soaked it all in. So now, it's time to squeeze the sponge and share some of what I've learned on this journey, particularly as it pertains to fitness and aging.

At 64, I'm not old. And more importantly, I feel about 40. I'm locked into a holding pattern right there, and I'm not alone thinking this way. That's why I'm writing this book. I know there are a lot of us out there who feel the same. I want to share my experiences to help others keep moving forward. I want you to forge your own new path—outside.

I'm part of a new movement within my generation—some call us anti-agers. We're baby boomers who don't view getting older or a few grey hairs as the end or the decline of anything. In some ways, we're just getting started: learning new skills, starting new careers and businesses, keeping up with technology, discovering new music, hiking, running, biking, golfing, surfing, weight-lifting, skiing, swimming, skydiving, tennis, and so on—same as always.

A lot of us have felt this way for decades, as you can see by the number of people who continue to enjoy the active lives they've lived thus far. It just never occurred to us to slow down. We're still planning for a future of unlimited possibilities, always wondering what's around the corner or just over the horizon. Many of us fully expect to see our great-grandchildren. Some of us will make it to age 100 and are planning for thirty or forty more years of good living and continuous exploration and learning.

Just a generation ago, this attitude and this level of physical and career activity were unheard of in people in their 50s, 60s, or older. There was the cultural expectation that aging meant slowing down, taking it easy, retiring, getting sick or injured, moving into a retirement community, and eventually fading away out of sight on Medicare and Social Security. This is not for us.

I was recently mentioned in a *Psychology Today* article about risk-takers, called "Lust for Life" (Carter 2020). That phrase is exactly the way we anti-agers feel. I got that way by being outside, staying active, and walking uphill—a lot.

At an age when some of my peers are talking retirement, I've never worked harder, and slowing down is the last thing on my mind. I have three jobs. All are demanding and require me to be on the front edge of multiple business categories. I get the opportunity to work happily with people young enough to be my grandkids. I can continue to work at this pace because I am fit, energetic, sharp as ever, and looking to the future with great optimism.

Read on and begin to defy aging. Learn to dismiss outdated thinking about getting older and how to join the ranks of anti-agers as we rewrite the rules for living longer lives.

And by the way, along my journey, all that plane, trail, tent, and hut time gave me time to think, ponder it all, and reconnoiter the world. I wasn't searching for it, but along the way, I found the fountain of youth.

Hint: it's hiking.

See you on the trails,

*Martin*

# INTRODUCTION

## My Wish for You

*If I knew I was going to live this long,*
*I'd have taken better care of myself.*

— MICKEY MANTLE

My wish is that this book will inspire you to be proactive about taking better care of yourself.

I want you to take charge of the way you age and make yourself more resistant to physical and cognitive decline. I want you to be better able to fight off sickness and recover faster if you should become sick. And I want to motivate you to share these ideas and advice broadly with your family and friends, and especially your parents. I hope my words will inspire you in many ways, but specifically:

**Be Active.** Go for long walks in nature, in the neighborhood, or anywhere your feet take you. Exercise, hike up a hill, or even climb a mountain. Use these physical movements to find a path to a happier, healthier, longer life.

We are going to live a long time beyond the traditional retirement age of 65. Our quality of life during those years depends a great deal on being healthy, fit, and active in both body and brain. While I could not save my own parents from a premature decline, you can take action now to slow down and even reverse the aging process.

**Get Outside.** Walking, especially uphill and hiking, takes fitness to the next level. You'll gain physical as well as mental strength and find calm in the outdoors that will recharge your brain and make you less susceptible to illness and more productive and creative in life.

**Get Off the Beaten Path.** I hope my experiences will motivate you to broaden your horizons and experience the awe that is readily available if you look for it. You might even learn how to better face adversity, stress, or depression, to deal with it, and walk right over the top of it.

**It's Not Too Late.** Finally, let me assure you of this: whatever fitness level or age, you can do this, and it will make a difference. Taking the first steps towards fitness, no matter how small, will have immediate, perceptible, and measurable physical and cognitive benefits. You will be taking steps toward a happier, healthier, longer life. And as your fitness level increases, every aspect of your life will improve. Yes, that's the way this works.

I'm not going to try to convince you to climb mountains. I'm going to try to motivate and ease you into walking more, then adding some uphill, then hiking, and then trekking farther, but only if you are up for it. Take small steps, and at any point, you can decide when you've reached your personal goal. There are big returns every step of the way.

One last thing: even though this book is called *Secrets of Aging Well,* frankly, these are only secrets because far too many people aren't aware of them. I'm merely trying to help make them less secret. It's never too late to learn them.

I've organized the book into four sections where I explain what I've seen and learned. My goal is to be your guide as you start your own journey to fitness. You can leave behind any trepidation or fear of the unknown as you take the first step on this unknown trail. I'll be with you to point out hazards as well as the beauty around us. For those of you who are already "gym fit" but are ready for a change, I'll show you what you've been missing and how much fun you're going to have outside.

## **SECTION 1:** The Fountain of Youth

In this section, you'll discover that the fountain of youth isn't in a miracle drug or good genes. It's hidden in the choices you make every day. As we start to live longer than any other generation, it's especially important that we challenge ourselves to make choices that keep us mentally and physically fit. This section helps you understand how to change your thinking, which results in changed behavior.

## **SECTION 2:** Lessons Learned Over 100,000,000 Uphill Steps

Here's the bad news/good news section. The bad news is that I've done lots of research, and it's time us to wake up. Studies show people are becoming inactive, sedentary, and unfit. These behaviors increase health risks, cost society a lot of money, and worse, decrease our quality of life. Medicine isn't the solution. The good news is that by being fit and healthy, we become our own preventive healthcare plan.

## **SECTION 3:** Fitness You Can't Get in a Gym

True fitness challenges your mind and body, and that's something you can only find outside. This section looks at the benefits of getting outdoors and pushing yourself beyond your comfort zone.

It encourages you to keep moving forward by finding your own peak or goal. The benefits are physical and cognitive—getting outside not only improves your fitness but actually improves brain function as well.

## SECTION 4: Get Outside

Here is where it all comes together, ranging from the how-tos of hiking to becoming the best version of yourself. In this section, we start with small steps—just getting outside for a walk—and then go through how you progress to longer and more challenging adventures. There are lots of tips—what you need to get started, how you find the right places, and how to plan and pack. And we talk about the importance of always having a goal—no matter what your "mountain" is.

## You Can Do This!

Throughout the book, you're going to see pictures and stories of people I've met along the way on trails and in hiking groups. These are not tales about famous mountain climbers or endurance athletes sponsored by gear companies and energy drinks. They're people like you. People who discovered, for varying and sometimes very personal reasons, that getting outside, into nature, and walking uphill can open up a whole new life of more energy, more confidence, better health, and less stress that will help you in every facet of your life. I've put many more of them on the book's website at **GetOutside.online**.

I've been surprised and pleased by how many people have been not only eager to share their stories, but eager to see others succeed on the same journey. It's been especially fascinating to see how many people in their 60s, 70s, and 80s discovered hiking late in life and used it as the catalyst for a happier, healthier, longer life.

These stories are absolutely heroic in my view. And you can do it too. If you think you can't, try thinking about it this way: *you can't do it ... yet*. By the end of this book, I think you will see what I mean and why.

So, yes, you can do this too.

Add "yet" to any statement about what you feel you can't do.

---

> *"A hero is an ordinary individual who finds the strength to persevere and endure in spite of overwhelming obstacles."*
>
> – Christopher Reeve

---

SECTION 1

# The Fountain of Youth

# 1

# EVERYTHING STARTS WITH A SINGLE STEP

*The journey of a thousand miles begins with one step.*

— LAO TZU

A long hike is a near-perfect analogy for life. One foot in front of the other, a series of single steps, over and over again. Some steps are uphill, some steps down, some are easy, some hard, sometimes you slip and skid, sometimes you coast downhill, occasionally you fall on your face. The truth is, no matter what comes your way, all you have to do is put one foot in front of the other, again and again, and you'll get through it.

But before any of us can start a long hike, we need to take the first step, and that's where this section begins—with a single step towards change. We're going to look at how to improve the trajectory of your life, how to delay the decline, and how to live a longer, happier, healthier life. We're going to discover that the fountain of youth isn't in a miracle drug or good genes. You'll find it when you make the choice to take a single step forward toward better health and fitness.

Although that step is likely to challenge you, you're going to do it anyway. That first step will put you on a journey that will keep you mentally and physically fit, and that is truly the fountain of youth.

## First Steps

Everyone, and I mean *everyone*, starts at the bottom—as a neophyte, a newbie, an amateur, a greenhorn, a tenderfoot, an apprentice, a beginner.

Formula One race car drivers, 747 pilots, Olympic athletes, elite high-altitude mountaineers, concert pianists—all began as novices. So, there is no need to be anxious about starting something new. As you begin your path toward better health, fitness, and longevity, simply focus on the first step. Everything else follows from that first action.

The best part of focusing on a single step is that there is a high

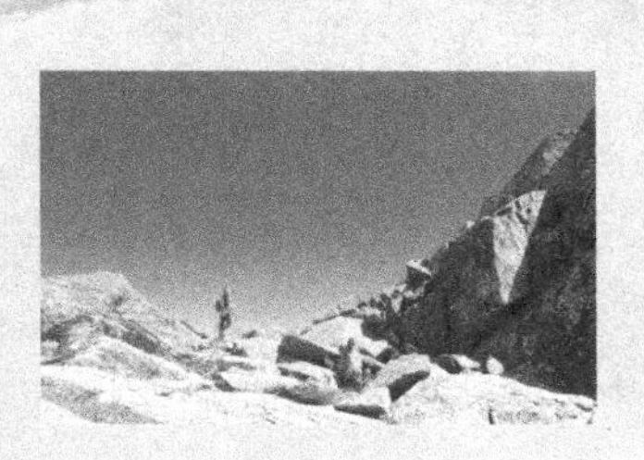

*Hiker on Mount Monadnock, New Hampshire*

"You must head up into the high country of the soul, into wild and uncharted regions and track down that elusive prey."

– *Wild at Heart*, John Eldredge

This is not easy to do. You're going to encounter obstacles. You're going to experience bad weather and setbacks. Some bumps and bruises are inevitable, as are discomfort, exhaustion, and so on.

So what? Such is life. You deal with it. You stare up at that obstacle and break it down into little pieces, one step at a time. You suck it up and find that pot of gold, that elusive moment, that special place. Or you never take a risk. You sit at home wondering what might have been and never experience the joy that is possible from these endeavors.

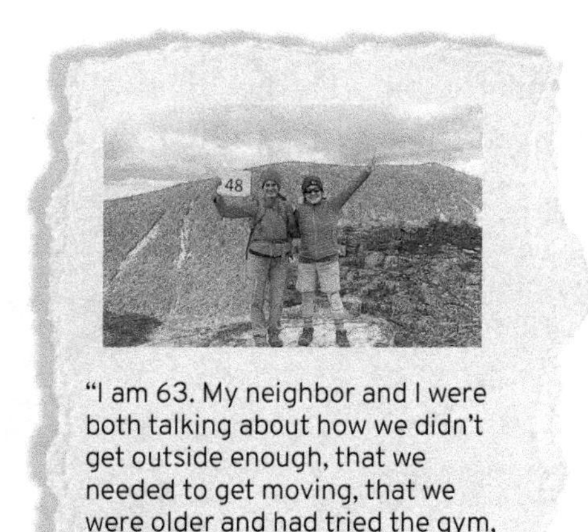

"I am 63. My neighbor and I were both talking about how we didn't get outside enough, that we needed to get moving, that we were older and had tried the gym, so we just hiked up local Mount Monadnock. Then, we did a few more and I was hooked."

– Andrea Mcgill O'rourke (with Cathy Carabello), New Hampshire

probability you will succeed. It's only one step, and you know you can do that. Instead of thinking about the immensity of the entire task before you, which can be daunting, you merely have to take that one baby step.

This works for every goal. Do you want to lose weight? Focus on losing that first pound or two. Do you want to hike a particular five-mile uphill trail? Start by walking a mile on flat ground. Those small steps add up.

No matter how big the challenge, no matter how long the trail, no matter how tough the problem, or how high the mountain, big challenges need to be looked at as a series of smaller problems. Breaking them into individual steps and smaller, manageable pieces add up (surprise!) and, over time, can result in seriously big accomplishments.

For instance, losing one pound per week, a manageable goal, can become 50 pounds total by the end of one year—a life-changing accomplishment. Or increasing the distance you walk by 5 percent a week every week turns a one-mile walk into almost 3.5 miles by the end of six months. If you increase your walking distance by 10 percent per week (which is very possible), you're suddenly walking 10 miles by the end of 6 months. Walking 10 miles is seriously good fitness. Small steps add up to big accomplishments.

Along the way, there will certainly be setbacks. Try not to worry too much about these. They are normal and to be expected. During my comeback periods, my first steps were fraught with setbacks. At times, my setbacks felt pretty overwhelming. When I started feeling that way, I would go back to my single-step thinking and keep moving forward. Eventually, I learned to recognize setbacks not as the end of the line but rather as challenges to be overcome.

My only semi-serious hiking injury came at a time when I was just getting back into hiking after a decade of exile, so I can't exactly say I was in the best shape. It was a simple slip, the result of inattentiveness. I was actually standing on the summit of Mount Washington in New Hampshire. It was pouring rain and one of the few times in my life I hadn't planned to hike to the top. Yes, I took the famed auto road because I was with some friends who were not hikers. The experienced international mountaineer (me) climbed onto a boulder to point out some mountain features when I slipped on the wet rock, landed on my elbow, dislocating it, with a hairline fracture of my forearm.

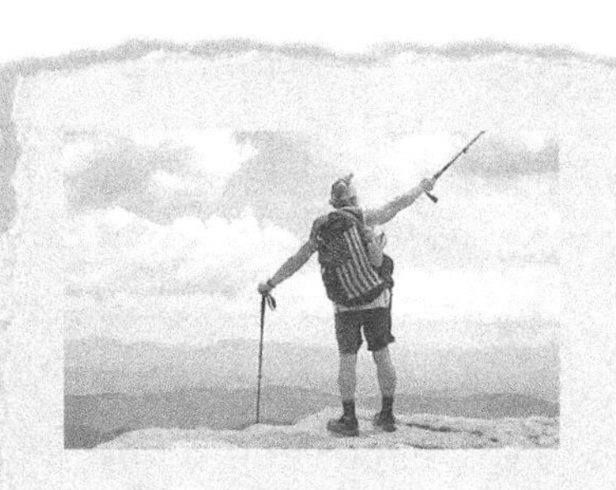

*Tim Andrew*

Tim Andrew, a retired firefighter from Connecticut, now living in the mountains of New Hampshire: "I had never hiked before, and I noticed hikers coming out of a trail at a rest stop in Vermont. I was a biker at a motorcycle rally, and asked one, 'What are you guys doing?' A woman answered, 'We're hiking the Appalachian Trail.' Now, I'm hiking the thing myself! I left on my 65th birthday. I discovered that anyone could hike, even long distances. It's pretty great not to watch all the negative news on TV every day."

This was my first baby step back on the very mountain that had started my mountaineering career, and it resulted in a broken arm! I could have interpreted this as a sign that I was not meant to get back into hiking and climbing, that I was too old or out of shape. Instead, I wore the setback as a badge. It was a learning experience that I should not let my guard down. I wasn't paying attention, even though I knew the rocks were wet. Basically, I wasn't taking proper precautions. The fall was not hiking's fault. It was my own fault, so I just needed to keep going and take the next step.

---

*"It does not matter how slowly you go as long as you do not stop."*

**– Confucius**

---

## Moving Forward

Once you've taken the first step, it's important to keep taking steps forward and challenging yourself. The best way to do that is to gradually increase the difficulty of what you're doing.

At each new level, you reset back to novice. A really competent walker and fitness buff who has never hiked is a novice again when they take the leap to hiking. They're learning new skills, a new mindset, and a different type of fitness. The beauty of this is that it happens over and over again at each level.

An experienced hiker and trekker, making the leap to climbing, goes through the same process. Then again, if that climber goes from climbing rocks to climbing snow and ice, or if they go from the famed 14,000-foot peaks in the Rockies to the daunting +20,000-foot peaks in the Himalayas. Each progression involves a reset to zero and another series of new first steps.

Let's go back to Mount Washington in New Hampshire. I had proven to myself in my early teens that I could climb it in the summer and winter. To accomplish this, I took numerous baby steps to prepare. I had honed my skills by hiking and camping on easier, more accessible mountains. I started out at High Rock State Park in Naugatuck, Connecticut. Then, I hiked Bear Mountain in the northwest corner of Connecticut and finally Mount Monadnock in New Hampshire.

I needed to climb other things and try other routes as I prepared for Mount Washington. Each step of the way, I increased the degree of difficulty to prepare myself for bigger challenges. Eventually, my youngest brother John and I climbed Mount Washington together via the hardest route. We went up the Huntington Ravine trail, which is listed as the most difficult in the White Mountains. It was a great climb and easier than we expected.

Once I knew I could do that route, I went back a few months later and climbed it solo. I began to realize what I could accomplish, what I could safely do, and what I needed to work on to improve. I also saw what others were doing and what was possible. After that climb, it all started to make sense—one small step after another gets you where you want to go. It's a natural progression. **Aim a little higher, push yourself a little harder, take a bit more risk, repeat as often as necessary, and you'll make progress.**

It's not a coincidence that the world opened up to me once I fully assimilated this lesson. I applied the skills I learned on the mountain to other parts of my life, especially business. I learned to be confident and not fear setbacks or failures. I learned when to take calculated risks and when to be bold and fearless. I learned to aim high. Even though at that point I had never climbed anything considered significant (or even out of New England), I had set a strong foundation. Being brave enough to take those first steps and to keep moving forward was the basis for everything else.

As more people come to know the benefits of getting outside, taking those first steps, and when ready, hiking up hills, they can experience this incredible life-altering, health-altering, mind-altering journey for themselves.

So many people have found the strength to get up and get outside. To experience the satisfaction of going over and through barriers that were holding them back, and into a realm of enhanced fitness and happier, healthier, longer lives.

Remember, if your boot slips on the first step, shrug it off and keep going—more on this later.

---

*"You keep putting one foot in front of the other, and then one day you look back and you've climbed a mountain."*

**– Tom Hiddleston**

---

# 2

# I'VE BEEN DOWN, BUT I GOT UP

*Fall seven times. Stand up eight.*

— ZEN PARABLE

In my thirties, I was an extremely fit, world-class climber. In my forties, I fell into a trap. I immersed myself in stressful work with extensive travel and too much expense account dining. Little by little, I was taking steps in a direction that made me inactive, overweight, and lazy. I lost my physical skills.

Frankly, this is not an isolated problem. Our population has become sedentary and less fit. As a result, there's an obesity and diabetes epidemic that inevitably leads to larger epidemics of heart, joint, brain, and other problems. Combined, these health issues will bankrupt families and even society if we do not solve it.

Luckily, in my 50s, I figured it out. I got fit again and got smart about aging. My fitness reboot helped me understand the danger we're facing as a society by neglecting our health. We need to focus on fitness options that are accessible, economical, and behaviorally possible for many. Getting outside, walking, and hiking check all the boxes.

My forties were a period when, despite the outward appearance of professional success, I was extremely miserable. My life was consumed by work and excessive plane, train, automobile, and hotel time. Over the course of a decade, my active lifestyle of hiking and climbing dwindled to an occasional activity. I worked out less, yet still paid for a gym membership I barely used. I sat in endless traffic in New York City, Chicago, and Los Angeles or crept along on Amtrak. To make matters worse, I took on a couple of high-stress, high-risk corporate roles where expense account dining was the norm.

Ironically, one of those roles was on the executive team at the world's largest fitness company. Even then, when I had a complete fitness club literally attached to my office and a big, often empty lap pool in the basement, I never seemed to find enough time to work out and practice what I was preaching to the world. The result was that little by little, over the course of a decade, I added an extra fifty pounds to my once lean-and-mean physique.

All my adventuring in high places of the world was replaced with excessive restaurant dining four or five times a week, a boatload of stressful problems to solve, 24/7 email, and endless texting from employees, clients, bankers, and board members. I'd like to say I felt it happening, but I didn't.

It was a slow process where I eventually found that walking uphill, once nearly effortless, was a struggle. My few feeble attempts to hike even small hills during this time revealed my physical condition was deteriorating and compromised. From my office in Santa Monica, I could see the famous Hollywood Hills. They lured me into a pedestrian hike up Runyon Canyon, a popular dog-walking spot with winding, well-trodden trails. I was quickly out of breath and tired. My lack of fitness was exposed, and I felt like a total embarrassment to myself. Instead of taking this as a wake-up call, I just became grumpier than usual at this revelation.

I was also experiencing sleep problems that were made even worse by frequent major time zone switches between New York and Hong Kong, Los Angeles to London to Dubai, and the ceaseless JFK to LAX back and forth. No amount of rest seemed to matter. And then, driving home from the airport after a long international trip, I got run off the highway by a truck changing lanes. Pushed up and over a guard rail, I took out a highway sign, tore all four wheels off the car, and came to rest in the center median. Fortunately, I was not injured (thank you Volvo), but I believe I might have avoided the accident completely if I was better rested and sharper. My sleep deprivation turned out to be another wake-up call.

At the same time, my parents' health began to decline. My father, once a superhero firefighter, retired early and in seemingly good health. But a major heart attack at age 65 set him back. An ensuing kidney failure led to a slow health decline that was painful to watch, especially because it could have been avoided. His superhero exterior masked a decaying, clogged cardiovascular system from a lifelong smoking habit, poor diet, and not enough exercise.

Then, my mother, who had managed to quit smoking cold turkey at age 40, began an even longer and more painful deterioration courtesy of a COPD (emphysema) diagnosis. In addition to the awful downward spiral that goes with that, she fell getting out of bed, broke a hip, and contracted pneumonia.

My parents were utterly unselfish. They raised four kids and put us through college on blue-collar wages, never putting themselves first. Unfortunately, they also smoked cigarettes, didn't exercise enough, worked too hard, and retired too soon.

Even though they looked pretty good on the outside, they were both ticking time bombs on the inside, ones that went off in their early 60s.

More alarm bells went off in my head.

During this time, I recall my dad calling to tell me how proud he was to see one of my commercials airing on television. It was one I had masterminded for the fitness company I worked for, and he was watching it *during a session at the kidney dialysis center*. The irony was indeed completely lost on me at the time.

I started to think more about their health and what led up to their health issues. They both went into a decline that coincided almost exactly with their move into a retirement community in Florida. They spent the last years of their lives consumed by illness, hospitals, dialysis, and assisted living and missed out on at least a decade of travel, grandkids, friends, good times … life.

I wish I had been able to share with my parents the experience and knowledge I now have. Many of their health issues could have been prevented if we had been smarter about aging and made better lifestyle choices decades earlier. It has motivated me to try to

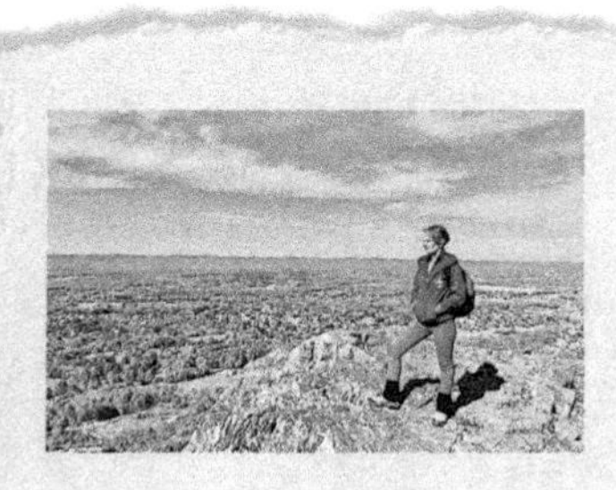

"I'm in my 60s. I hiked to the top of Mount Quandary in Colorado. Up until then, I had never seen a 360-degree view from a mountain peak. There are no words to describe the splendor. What a gift I received to be there. It was the hardest thing I ever did. It was exhilarating! It felt like every cell in my body was humming with life. Since that day four years ago, I have become an avid hiker and all my vacations have been in the hills, hiking and being in nature."

– Pat Mattas, Connecticut

help others avoid this same scenario and compelled me to write this book.

Frankly, my parents' experience is not an isolated problem. It's widespread in our aging population. People are becoming less active and eating poorly. As a result, there's an obesity and diabetes epidemic that inevitably leads to larger epidemics of heart, joint, brain, and other problems.

The only answer to this problem is fitness at a population level. Being fit and healthy benefits both individuals and society. To motivate people to live healthier lives, we need to listen to those alarm bells and make some important changes.

## I Rediscover Hiking

Eventually, those alarm bells turned into wailing sirens somewhere deep in my head. It took me a while to hear them, too long really. But finally, one perfect, crisp fall day, I dug out my hiking boots and dusty red backpack, filled it with about twenty pounds of gear and hiked about eight miles through the Connecticut hills. Nothing major. I moved very slowly. My heart was pounding, my thighs and calves were screaming, but, oh what a rush I got—the perfect primal act of one foot in front of the other, the deliberate uphill movement over uneven terrain, the utter simplicity of it. Even the aches and pains the next day were more like welcome old friends than an annoyance.

Just a single hike reminded me how much I loved it, how happy I was to be doing it again, and how lucky I was that my own poor lifestyle decisions had not resulted in something worse than getting a bit chunky. Luckily, as cranky and irritable as I had become, I still had my physical health, probably thanks to the latent effects of being so fit in my thirties and forties (this is called "dormant physiological reserve").

It took a few months of two to three good walks or hikes per week (and no more pizza or McDonald's) to get back in the groove. The more I walked, the more I felt like working out in the gym. I felt better. I even slept better. The spring in my step returned. My pace quickened over time, and the hills got bigger and steeper. Before long, the extra weight poured away, and I became more energetic and focused. My mood improved, as did my work productivity. I found the old me again—actually, an older and wiser version of the old me.

And it seems to be working. How do I know this?

Well, I just trekked 100 miles across Nepal to Mount Everest with a great group of other super-fit anti-agers. Two of them, in their 60s, have climbed Everest on multiple occasions. Last year, I raced up to the top of the Empire State Building for charity, wearing a 30-pound backpack. I'm on the tail end of summiting the 48 tallest peaks in New Hampshire. Forty of those excess fifty pounds are gone. Not only do I feel great, but after all the pounding those 100,000,000 steps have given me, I'm very happy to be 100 percent original—no replacement hips or knees and no medications.

I was down, but now I'm back up. If you feel down or unable to get yourself going, ***rest assured, you can do this***. I know this with certainty because I've been there. I've also talked with hundreds of people I've met along the way—on trails and in hiking groups. At some point, they've all been in the same spot where they weren't sure what to do. They discovered—as you'll see in their stories throughout the book—hiking is indeed the fountain of youth.

# 3

# HIKING IS THE FOUNTAIN OF YOUTH

*"We must all either rust out or wear out. Every one of us. I chose to wear out."*

— TEDDY ROOSEVELT

Rust out? No way. Rust is for old, broken-down, useless, inactive things. Damn it; we are none of those things. If you feel like you're headed in that direction, I want to get you straightened out: it's not too late to turn it around.

Fitness, especially the kind you can achieve outside by walking and then hiking, can slow down and even reverse the tide of aging.

Fit people get sick less. Fit people have bigger brains. Fit people spend less on healthcare. Fit people live longer. And hiking is possibly the best anti-aging activity there is. I think it's the fountain of youth.

I started hiking as a boy scout at age 12. My father was our scoutmaster, and he believed that hiking built strong bodies and developed a sense of self-reliance and confidence. It also encouraged an appreciation for the awesomeness of nature.

Because he was incapable of sitting still for very long, I think he also hoped hiking would give us some of that same energy.

My dad had been in the Army in the early 1950s and was stationed in Germany, not far from the Zugspitze, the country's highest mountain. Looking back, I now see how it influenced him to believe that hiking was his version of putting us through basic training and boot camp. No complaints there, he was right. Hiking was incredibly formative and, for me, became the norm. Excursions across the hills of New England were a regular feature throughout my teens and twenties. But it did not strike me as unique training until I was in my early thirties and had become an accomplished hiker and climber (in large part because of my early experiences in the mountains).

It was August 1992. While descending the upper slopes of Mount Washington in New Hampshire at a very rugged area known as the Rockpile, I was still well above treeline with three hours of steep, rugged downhill ahead. I was nearly 3,000 vertical feet from my car at the trailhead. The Rockpile is notorious for high winds and sudden weather changes that can kill an unprepared hiker, even in summer. While this was not a major climbing expedition, it was by no means an easy walk in the woods.

At the time, I was very fit and hefting a heavy backpack as part of my training for an upcoming climb of Mount Rainier, the massively glaciated peak in Washington State that is the breeding ground for more Everest guides and summiteers than anywhere else in the world. Mount Washington, the tallest peak in the Northeast, is an excellent training ground for these bigger mountains. During my twenties and thirties, it was not uncommon for me to climb it about ten times per year.

While moving down the Rockpile, I noticed far below me a solo hiker—actually, a trail runner before that was even a thing.

He was bounding uphill at an impressive pace and headed straight for me after cresting a feature known as Lion Head. When he got closer, I could see this was not a young man. In fact, the closer he got, the more I watched in disbelief as this lean runner, clearly old enough to be my grandfather, made his way toward me in shorts and sneakers, no backpack, and only a water bottle and trekking poles for equipment. He bounced from rock to rock with the confidence and balance of an acrobat.

This gentleman, I learned, was 75-years old, and I did not doubt that he was fitter than me. He pulled up and said hello. "How … how are you doing this?" was about all I could mutter in disbelief. "I've been running up this hill twice a week since I was younger than you, son. Keeps me young! Have a great day!" and he resumed his relentless uphill jog to the summit, 500 vertical feet above. As I descended, I kept looking over my shoulder to see how he was progressing, amazed that his pace had not slacked at all on his way to the summit.

Mind totally blown.

I didn't know it at the time, but it was a turning point in my life—a revelation, both humbling and inspirational. I never imagined it was possible to be that fit at that age. My own grandfather could not

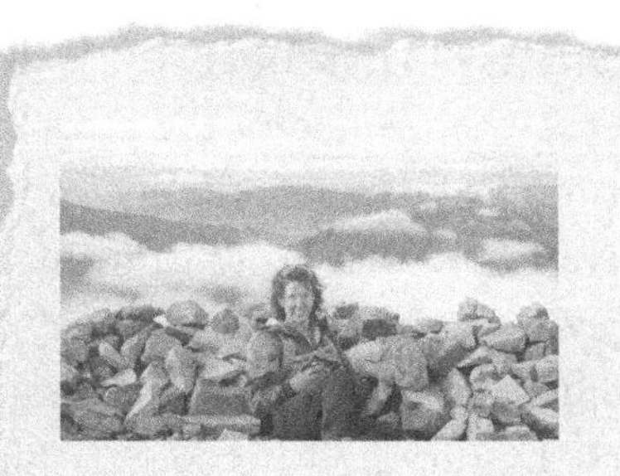

"I'm extremely afraid of heights. And that kind of led me to be a mountaineer. Just because I didn't want my mind to control my whole being, my soul. So, I decided to control my mind. I learned how to set my fear to the side. And so, to me that's the fountain of youth. Pushing yourself beyond your limits. And being able to put that fear aside and move forward, in spite of it."

– Lisa Veraldi, Colorado

do that, and no one I knew had a grandfather who could do that. It got me thinking, "Hey, maybe I can still be doing this at his age!" and "I wonder how I can train for that?" Then, I had a lot of questions: "Is hiking what enables this kind of physical performance? Or is it exercise in general? Or is it being outdoors a lot? Maybe hiking is the fountain of youth?"

Now, I know the answers: yes, it is hiking. I had indeed found the fountain of youth.

## What Makes Hiking the Fountain of Youth?

What I've learned since that day on Mount Washington in 1992 is that the physical act of hiking creates a potent and unique positive effect on the human body and, more importantly, on the brain. The combined benefits are the result of multiple factors, including:

**Bursts of High Intensity.** Walking up a steep trail with a pack on your back is one of the most intense workouts you can have. Short bursts of high-intensity exercise spaced out over the day are known to produce rapid gains in fitness levels. They also increase longevity over the long term. The beauty of a hike is that you're able to completely control your heart rate throughout the course of a day simply by varying your speed. The faster you go, the harder your heart works. Need a break? Slow down or stop to catch your breath. Then pick up the pace again to boost the heart rate. This means you can experience many instances of high-intensity training mixed in with moderate or relaxed paces as needed.

Hiking is not a race, so you can adjust your pace as needed. This up-and-down pattern of exercise intensity is extremely effective at building heart rate variability. Heart rate variability is the difference between your resting heart rate and your maximum heart rate under intense exercise.

With better fitness, your resting heart rate goes down, and your maximum heart rate goes up. The greater the difference between the two, the stronger and more resilient your heart.

**Weight-Bearing.** When astronauts return from an extended stay in space, they often find they have lost muscle and bone mass. This is because when weightless, the body is hardly stressed at all. As a result, it adapts to the lack of stress that gravity normally provides by essentially shrinking.

Here on earth, we can produce the opposite effect. The more weight-bearing exercise you do, the more your body adapts to it by growing stronger muscles and denser bones.

Hiking is a phenomenal weight-bearing exercise, and it triggers numerous physiological benefits. Every step you take helps to build a stronger skeletal system. Stronger bones permit stronger muscles and are much more resistant to breaks.

There's also the fact that exercising your legs is by far the best way to create full-body benefits. Your large leg muscles will act as a secondary pump for your circulatory system that boosts the efforts of your heart and makes more blood and oxygen available to the rest of your body, especially your brain.

**What Goes Up Must Come Down.** If you're a fan of the Stairmaster at the gym, you already know how great a workout that can be. But here's a surprise: downhill is just as good for you and, in some ways, even better.

Though hiking downhill is easier on you aerobically, it actually engages a different set of muscles and in a different way. Uphill uses concentric contractions of the muscles; downhill uses eccentric contractions. In a nutshell, this means the weight-bearing effect is intensified because you expend an incredible amount of energy resisting the force of gravity to decelerate your body and prevent falling forward. This process also engages your core muscles to help keep you upright.

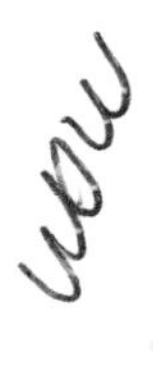

Every step of a long descent creates powerful contractions of the leg muscles that are barely used when running on flat ground or hiking uphill. When you hike downhill, you actually use up to three times more energy compared to uphill. There's very powerful fitness training happening on the downhill.

**Engages Your Brain.** Every step on uneven terrain involves a complex interplay between your eyes, your brain, and your muscles to keep you upright, to keep you moving, and to prevent you from falling. You've heard of hand-eye coordination that is so important in many sports? Well, hiking requires a significant amount of foot-eye coordination, which is far more intense for your brain.

A five-mile hike is about 10,000 steps, and the same is true for a five-mile walk on a treadmill. However, all steps are not created equal.

On a treadmill, your brain switches to autopilot because it's flat and safe, and you barely need to think about foot placement. On uneven terrain, like hiking outdoors, those 10,000 steps mean 10,000 separate calculations your brain has to make to keep you from falling and tripping while moving forward, upward, and downhill.

This is exponentially more engaging than toiling along on a treadmill where the surface is predictable. This particular feature of hiking—the high level of neural activity it requires—creates denser neural pathways. Think of these pathways as strands of connected brain cells. This is how your brain controls your body, and the more you use it like this, the more neural pathways you create. The result over time is a brain that is much more resilient to cognitive decline.

**Soothes Your Mind.** Not only is the sunshine beneficial, but the sights and sounds of a natural environment (birds chirping, ocean waves, running streams and waterfalls, wind through the trees, thunderstorms, etc.) have broad, positive effects on mood, reduce anxiety and stress, increase creativity and attention span, improve the immune system, and much more. These benefits offset the daily stress and tension of city life and can cure burnout.

Birdsong, in particular, has a wonderful soothing effect on the human brain. That's because eons ago, primitive humans knew that when the birds were singing, there were no predators in the area. That's still hardwired into our brains. More birdsong mean less burnout.

**Natural Vision Improvement.** If you spend a significant amount of time indoors staring at a TV screen, computer, tablet, or mobile phone, you are not using the full capabilities of your eyes. In essence, your eye muscles are not getting a full workout, and they can atrophy.

When you frequently go outside and look at the world around you, your eyes dart around and move naturally to guide you through your movements. This needs to occur regularly to keep those muscles flexible and in command of the full range of motion.

When you go outside, you look in all directions (forward, sideways, and up) as you focus on your surroundings. You also engage your depth perception abilities, and you see in three dimensions, instead of a flat-screen.

This, in turn, enables the eye muscles to loosen up, remain flexible, and to use the full range of motion that they are designed for.

**Major Calorie Burn.** Compare hiking to walking on a flat treadmill at two miles per hour. A treadmill walk burns 170 calories per hour walking flat. Set at the same speed and a mild 15 percent incline, you would burn 448 calories. Hiking is often steeper than 15 percent and may include carrying the weight of a backpack, which makes the calorie burn significantly better. A backpack also increases the weight-bearing benefits of hiking and further strengthens your skeletal system. ***A steep uphill hike with a heavy pack can burn 750 to 1,000 calories per hour.***

So, if getting leaner is something you desire or if you want to rid yourself of excess body fat, there are few activities that can do it quite as well as hiking. Let's review the benefits:

- Bigger lungs and more endurance
- A solid cardiovascular system with an indestructible heart that keeps your brain and muscles at their best
- Improved eyesight
- Stronger, thicker bones
- Sharper thinking and improved creativity
- Springy, strong leg muscles
- A solid core that will keep you well balanced and impervious to serious harm if you fall

More importantly, don't you want all these seemingly different systems to work together in harmony, enabling you to move about the world with purpose, energy, and confidence? (Greville 2017)

Hiking accomplishes this synergy in ways that are hard to replicate in a gymnasium or a fitness club alone. For these reasons, it is possibly the best anti-aging activity out there, and why I believe it to be the fountain of youth.

Collecting rust? No way.

# 4

# CHANGE YOUR THINKING: YOU'RE NOT OLD

*How old would you be if you didn't know how old you are?*

— SATCHEL PAIGE

Satchel Paige was a professional baseball player known for his exceptionally long career. He played from 1926 until 1965 when he retired at age 47. Playing professional baseball at age 47—two generations ago—is the equivalent of playing in your 60s today. In a profession where the average career lasts about five years, and retirement typically occurs in your late twenties, Paige was generations ahead of his time, an outlier in the 99.9th percentile.

Truthfully, we need to adopt his attitude that age is as much a state of mind as it is a number. We must change the way we think about aging because there is a heck of a lot more longevity in the world now. This longevity introduces a number of issues into the equation. Think about these questions:

1. How will you afford to live during a 30- to 40-year retirement period?
2. Will your pension plan last for a 30- to 40-year retirement?
3. Will you be productive and active during those years of retirement, or inactive and an expensive drain on your savings, your family, and the healthcare system.

We've all heard that you are as young as you feel. The truth is you can feel more youthful and defy aging by being fit. Thankfully, the results of a recent survey show our attitudes toward "old age" are indeed changing. According to the American Society of Gerontologists, here's how to categorize your age:

- 45 to 64 is considered middle age.
- 65 to 74 is young old.
- 75 to 84 is categorized as old.
- 85 to 94 is categorized as old-old (but I believe that will be subject to additional modification as we continue to redefine our perception of age).
- 95 plus is called oldest old (and happens to be the fastest-growing age group of all).

This categorization would have been inconceivable in 1920 when the global life expectancy was 29 years old.

So, let's say it directly: if you're under 75, you're not old, so don't refer to yourself that way. If you're over 75, there's a lot you can do to change the trajectory of how you age by thinking, living, appearing, and acting much younger, so you're not really old either. And this phenomenon is only going to increase in the future. Even if you were not fit in your 40s or 50s, there are tremendous benefits and many upsides to getting fit in your 60s and 70s. It's never too late.

---

*"Getting old is a fascinating thing. The older you get, the older you want to get."*

**– Keith Richards**

---

We see evidence across the country and across the world that redefining how we label and think about age is already happening. **Active agers are continuing to lead vigorous and productive lives and are reshaping the way the world thinks about aging.** They're not prepared to give up active lifestyles, and they're definitely not prepared to go gently into that good night.

But changing attitudes are one thing. Changing behavior and taking action are what matters, and it would be great to see substantive progress in behavioral elements that give people the ability to be proactive about the way they age.

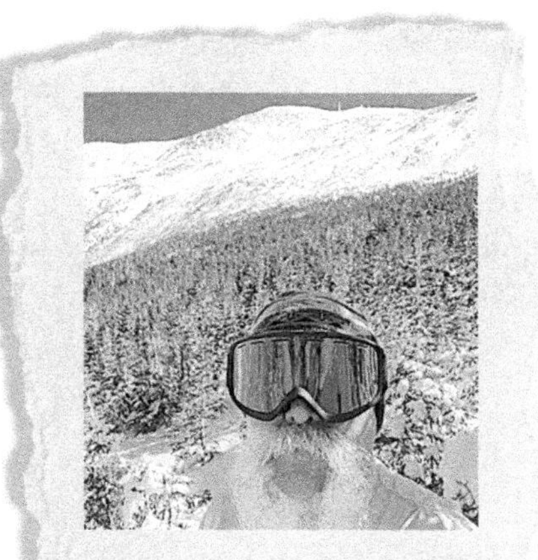

"When I turned 61, I decided to become more adventurous. I have found, when I go out and hike, there's a joyful peace in it all. And, while it can be difficult to actually start a hike, there is a true joy in completing it. A great sense of accomplishment and you feel good about yourself as a person. I will continue to hike for as long as I am healthy enough to continue. The simple joy of being out there far exceeds any discomfort that one runs into while hiking."

– Ralph Jesseman.
New Hampshire

## Changed Thinking Changes Behavior

If you still think you're old, you most likely just need to change the way you think. If you don't think you're old, that mindset is a highly persuasive thing that is likely to encourage you to behave younger in all facets of your life. It will give you the optimism you need to think ahead and plan, not for retirement, but to continue living the way you've always lived. I so wish my own progenitors had not given in to outdated ideas about aging.

My grandfather retired at 50 with health problems, and my father retired at age 65 only to have his health problems begin. In both their cases, smoking created those health problems. But it was also their mindset, thinking they were old, worn out, and finished. They felt retirement was a worthy goal, an achievement to be experienced as soon as possible. I watched as the whole retirement mentality kicked in, and these once active and virile men slowed down. They sat more, never exercised, and slid into a premature decline. You quite probably have a similar story in your family.

Sadly, my father's decline hastened my mother's. She not only slowed down, but she also became his principal caregiver, adding a whole new, all-consuming stressful element to her life. She started acting older, behaving as if she were at least 10 or 20 years older than her chronological age, and that scenario is all too common. Women tend to live longer than men and are more natural caregivers. Oftentimes, if a man gets sick first, his wife bears much of the burden. The impact of that completely changes the trajectory of both lives.

There are also increasing numbers of people whom researchers are calling the sandwich generation. This group is comprised of healthy people between the ages of 40 and 70, who are both raising their children and caring for their failing parents. The economic and emotional cost of that is practically incalculable and quite destructive.

Incidentally, I expect that women will be the ones who will quite rightly prod their husbands to get up off the couch and start moving. They have done the math on this and figured out that if they do not prod their couch potato into activity, they're going to get stuck being a caregiver instead of living an active, independent life.

That kind of downhill slide is not for me. I have no interest in being an expensive burden to my family or to the healthcare system if I can avoid it.

Instead, I want to follow people my age and older who really push the limits of what is possible. Satchel Paige was a start, but I'm quite inspired by people like Diana Nyad, who at age 64 swam the 75 miles from Florida to Cuba. I'm with Dale "Greybeard" Sanders, who at age 84 hiked the entire 2,180 miles of the Appalachian Trail from Georgia to Maine. And Bob Becker, who at age 70 ran the 292-mile Badwater Double across Death Valley, the lowest point in the country, and up to the top of Mount Whitney, the highest point in California. And I'm in awe of Yuchio Muira, who at age 70 climbed to the summit of Mount Everest and then did it again at age 80.

I could go on and on with cases of people, friends, and family, who are defying age and living large lives well into their 80s. Hikers, in particular, exhibit age-defying qualities. A common comment I heard from the hundreds of people I've interviewed is, "I have no age when I hike." These people and their attitudes inspire me to keep seeking new challenges.

## Living with Longevity

The current aging population is a tidal wave that has only just begun. It's an unstoppable tectonic force that will reshape economies, industries, jobs, healthcare, and more. It's already taken on a name: The Longevity Economy.

Did you know that in 2046 the first of the baby boomers turn 100? There's going to be a lot of them. It's already the fastest-growing segment of the population. And it's a group that has reshaped the culture from its origins after World War II through the turbulent 1960s to the boom years of the '80s and '90s and will continue to do so as we enter the post-pandemic years after 2020. Mark my words, they will indeed reinvent the way we age.

It has been said that longevity is the great gift of the twentieth century. Our challenge now is to learn to live with it. I'm choosing to use whatever longevity I get to do things that are productive, useful, rewarding, and fun. I'd rather not rust out or fade away while I still have things to do.

Like many anti-agers, I believe I'm just entering my prime at age 64, and I think I have at least 20 more highly productive years to go before I start to slow down—maybe more. Maybe I will never retire and either drop dead at my desk (hopefully at age 101) or fall off a mountain somewhere (also hopefully at age 101).

Living well into your 80s, 90s, and above 100 is totally off-the-map, uncharted territory. But that's the way it is with every new thing. Eventually, uncharted territory becomes comfortable terrain. The mountains and hills I regularly hike were once unmapped, unknown, wild, and scary. Now, they are not. That's the way it will be with aging, too. Let's redraw the map for how to do this.

---

*"Age is no barrier. It's a limitation you put on your mind."*

**– Jackie Joyner-Kersee**

---

# 5

# LONGEVITY CHANGES THE RETIREMENT EQUATION

*I see all these old people who don't have anything to do but eat, drink and sleep. I will never stay "retired" because that's such a finality that I don't want it to be part of my life. I'll work till they throw me in a box.*

— MARIO ANDRETTI

Not only are you most likely too young to retire, but why would you want to anyway? You'll age faster and possibly run out of money too soon. At 60 years old, you've likely only lived two-thirds of your life. What are you going to do with that remaining third? Go to the beach? Play golf? Binge-watch Netflix?

I've come to the conclusion that most people drastically underestimate how much longer they're going to live. Too many people are buying into a generations-old standard and automatically assuming that somewhere in your 60s is the appropriate time to retire. I think that's because most people think they'll begin to fade in their late 60s or early 70s, that they're less useful and productive than they were when they were younger, and that the money will never run out.

But the way things are trending, we need to realize that making it to age 90 is quite probable, and that age 100 is possible.

So, if you look to the future with that in mind, why retire early? What can you do with all that longevity? Have you prepared for it? Can you afford to live that long? Not only are you probably way too young to retire, but why would you want to anyway?

Just like my 75-year-old trail runner encounter changed my thinking about aging, working with real estate magnates George and Ron Rubin really opened my eyes to the future of a much later retirement. I collaborated with them on a fitness project some years ago, while they were running Pennsylvania Real Estate Investment Trust, owners of more than 50 shopping malls and numerous fitness clubs. At ages 76 and 80, they were in the office every day, working out every lunchtime, and defying aging in a way that shaped my thinking about the future. Working with them was a genuine eye-opener about remaining productive and engaged. They are a bellwether of things to come, and I expect this will be more the norm going forward.

So is Klaus Obermeyer, the founder of the Obermeyer sports clothing company, still skiing well at age 100. "The first hundred years are behind me; now it's on to the next century … You have to keep exercising," he says. "Your health should be your number one priority. Your body carries your brain. If your body is healthy, then your brain has a chance to be healthy, too" (Averill 2020).

These stories were in sharp contrast to what I experienced at home. As I mentioned earlier, my parents retired at ages 60 and 58 to a retirement community in Florida and were eager to do so. This completely blows my mind because I'm older than that right now, and I cannot fathom it at all. They had a totally different mindset about work and retirement, and I'm certain it contributed to their premature, rapid aging.

Just a few years before that, my dad was driving me to the airport as I was leaving for the Swiss Alps. I was going to climb the Matterhorn again (I was 32, he was 57), and he asked, "Is this your last big climb, while you still can? Are you going to retire from all this?"

"While I still can?!" I fumed back at him. His view of aging was that I was getting too old, at age 32. I have to admit it's also probable that, as a parent, he was worried I would eventually manage to get myself killed on a mountain. This from a man who had spent the last 25 years as a fireman running into burning buildings and across rooftops, in full gear.

On the other hand, I was just about at my physical prime—probably hadn't even peaked yet—and his last-generation mindset wanted me to slow down and play it safe. I thought I was barely getting started.

We differed about what happens as you age. I wanted to fight it, keep going, and defy aging. He thought I should start to cut back, play it safe, and slow down.

## Longevity Changes the Equation

When life expectancy was short, it made a certain degree of sense to think about slowing down in your late 50s or early 60s to enjoy a few years of relaxation and live off your retirement savings and Social Security. Right? You paid into it, and now it's time to get it back and enjoy life before you die.

But now, not only is the culture different, but the mindset is changing, and the economics of aging is different. People are starting to understand how to live longer. People are starting to understand that the act of slowing down contributes to and accelerates the decline.

Lawyer, business coach, and fellow outdoor adventurer Walt Hampton, who actively hikes and climbs all around the world in his 60s, sums it up nicely: "It's a bit discouraging to see former partners and colleagues capitulate to age and hang it up."

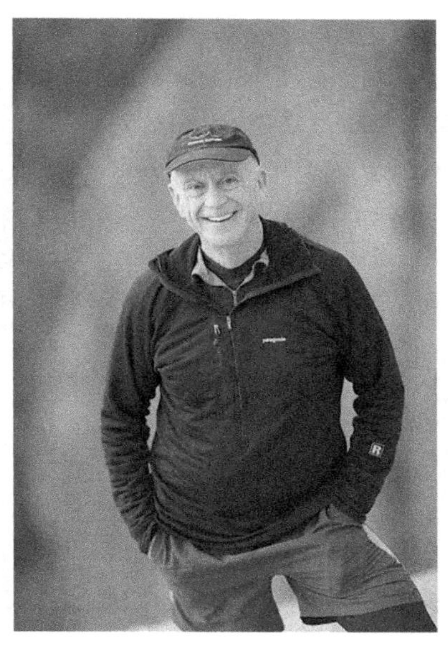

*Walt Hampton*

Experience and wisdom are invaluable, even in a world where the average age of a Google employee is 29, and ageism is rampant. In fact, the business world is just starting to realize that the expertise and wisdom of people in their 60s and 70s is a very valuable company and cultural asset.

People with many years of experience do not struggle with challenges and problems the same way inexperienced people do. We see things in the context of many years of problem solving and exposure to countless issues. And we've even developed an ability to see patterns and have insights that people with less experience cannot fathom.

All I can think of is how disappointing it is to see perfectly healthy and productive people decide they are done. Maybe it's not done consciously, but to enter into a retirement mindset, to stop thinking and stop moving, and to willingly slide down that curve of aging seems to me a terrible mistake, driven by the wrong attitude. More people need to open themselves to a new paradigm of aging.

Because really, what's the alternative? Golf? Boring. Plus, I'm lousy at it. Sitting on the beach in Florida? My parents did that; they aged 20 years in five. Growing old, spent, or dulled on the couch watching nonsense on TV—the slow decline into senility and death? No, that's definitely not for me. And it's not for a lot of others who are refusing to capitulate to age and illness the way our parents and grandparents did.

## Reboot Yourself

While many of us dream of a golden age of retirement, a 2016 study on early retirement found that it may be a risk factor for mortality. In fact, a prolonged working life may provide longevity and survival benefits. This study found that people who worked longer lived longer, a fact reflected in earlier longitudinal studies that found correlations between retirement and poor health. Researchers speculate that this is because working usually involves social interaction,

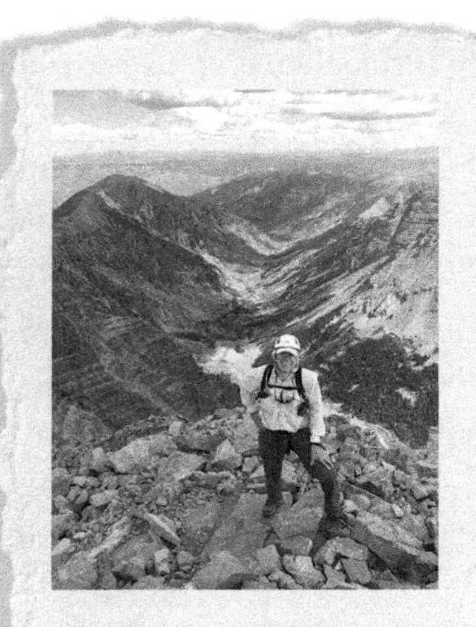

"I am 67. I started hiking when I retired. I will hike about 1,600 miles this year. I've had four knee replacements over the past ten years with the last one in 2016 and much more planned for 2020. I have two friends that I hike a lot with that are both 70. I have another very active friend who is 80."

– Tony Eichstadt, Colorado

movement, and a sense of purpose. Several studies have linked retirement with loneliness and depression (LaPonsie 2018).

But working long hours, year after year is not the answer either. Research shows that from mid-life onward, the sweet spot for health and longevity is working at a less intense pace and perhaps for fewer hours.

## Why You Shouldn't Retire Young

Even if you can retire, perhaps with a secure pension, or have to retire because you hate your job, don't retire, per se—find another avocation. Retrain, do something new. Retiring in the classic sense, to the beach, to the golf course, to the sofa, is the fastest way to age fast, lose your sharpness, and slide down that path to oblivion. Here are a few thoughts on the subject of why not to retire too soon:

1. You fade. If you stop moving and stop using your brain, you accelerate the downhill trajectory of aging.
2. It's lonely. Your social connections dwindle. Loneliness is a key factor in depression and advanced aging.
3. It's boring. You probably need something useful to do when the kids grow up and fly the coop
4. You have less anxiety about using up your retirement savings.
5. You're not done yet. If you're not satisfied and at peace with your life's work, use your remaining years to do something more, something new, something productive and useful. Volunteer, teach, mentor, invent, write. Put all those years to good use.

### Reasons to Keep Going

On the flip side, there are lots of reasons why you should keep going and doing. For starters, it helps you to maintain a positive outlook. Satisfaction with life goes way up with age if you feel useful, productive, and fully engaged.

Why not try hiking, trekking, mountain biking, or surfing? And with all that resulting newfound energy, maybe even create a startup company, or begin consulting and mentoring? There is an infinite number of ways to use your experience when you have the energy created by heightened fitness.

This is an overused example, but it's worthy of repeating: Colonel Sanders did not start Kentucky Fried Chicken until he was in his 60s. Granted, this was practically a miracle in the late 1950s and early 1960s (maybe as rare as Satchel Paige), but this is already fairly commonplace now and will be rampant over the next generation (Cheng 2019).

The good news for employers with an aging workforce? According to research from the Milken Institute's Center for the Future of Aging and the Stanford Center on Longevity, older employees take fewer sick days, show stronger problem-solving skills, and are more likely to be highly satisfied at work than their younger colleagues.

## Change Your Future

Get fit. Your brain will be sharper. Your energy and stamina will be higher. You'll look better, feel better, and be far more able to compete effectively in a marketplace that badly needs more 'adults in the room' and more of the wisdom that comes from experience.

And you won't be dependent on the kindness of strangers (or Social Security and Medicare), you won't fear running out of money too soon, and you'll keep building that nest egg for when retirement is a better option. Let's say not until at least the age of 80.

---

> *"You get in good shape, you feel good about your body and your spirit, and you enjoy life, so it's easy to look at things positively."*
>
> – **Klaus Obermeyer**, at age 100.

---

SECTION 2

# Lessons Learned Over 100,000,000 Uphill Steps

# 6

# AN INACTIVE, SEDENTARY, UNFIT, AGING POPULATION

*Sitting is the smoking of our generation.*

— NILOFER MERCHANT

Unfortunately, while active agers are redefining the way we age, they are still in the minority. Far too few people have adopted healthy, active lifestyles, so they enter their 50s and 60s already on the decline.

This is our generational and cultural problem in a nutshell: a massive, sedentary, aging, unfit, unhealthy, population bubble, and too few people who have adopted healthier lifestyles. There is going to be a very large price to pay for this if we do not become more proactive about the way we live and the way we age.

At the 2013 TED Conference, Silicon Valley strategist Nilofer Merchant reported that "people now sit for an average of 9.3 hours each day, compared with sleeping an average of 7.7 hours daily ... This growing inactivity is leading to greater obesity, which is a bigger health threat than smoking" (Merchant, *Harvard Business Review* 2014).

I'm certain this problem has increased since 2013. While I see signs that more people my age are taking steps to be more active and physically fit, the numbers do not lie. We need to make even more progress to help people live more active lives.

## Innovation?

Technology simplifies life. It's very cool stuff. Back in the 1970s, wired remote control televisions and radio-controlled garage door openers took care of simple daily tasks. Nowadays, Alexa and Siri use artificial intelligence to help us manage actions in our homes and beyond.

The trick is that these innovations are creating a culture of inactivity by allowing us to remain sedentary. Rather than getting up to change the television channel or open the garage door, we can adjust the thermostat, turn on the lights, start the car, order food, play games, go shopping, and so much more all without getting out of bed.

It seems like everything we create is encouraging more and more inactivity. There is now a whole generation of kids being taught to run their lives through voice-controlled apps on a screen. I'm hyperaware of this fact in my own life. I would bet that voice apps lull me into getting 500 to 2,000 fewer steps per day, maybe more. This is becoming a serious societal problem.

Add these innovations to a massive aging population that is living longer not because they are healthier or fitter, but because of surgery and medicine, and we have a problem. The problem is bigger than any mountain, bigger than any company or industry can handle, and bigger than any government or private healthcare program can fix.

Unless our society's behavior changes, more people will require expensive and ultimately unaffordable medical procedures or die prematurely because they can't access them. The implications of this simple fact are so wide-reaching and daunting it may feel easier to look the other way and do nothing. However, I believe much of this is preventable. But, before we talk about some of the solutions (like walking and hiking), let me terrify you with the facts.

## Metabolic Syndrome Is Rampant

You may not have heard the term metabolic syndrome, but it describes a collection of conditions that are the precursors to serious but preventable medical problems. These conditions include:

- Excess body fat in the midsection
- Increased blood pressure
- Increased cholesterol or triglyceride levels
- High blood sugar
- Sleep apnea

They can increase your risk of things like heart disease, stroke, and type 2 diabetes.

Most frequently, metabolic syndrome is the byproduct of the way inactive people live, and it is the root cause of many long-term and expensive medical problems. When these conditions begin to appear, it is a good idea to take action by starting to move more (getting outside, walking more, or hiking).

If you are overweight or obese, you probably have metabolic syndrome. If you have diabetes, you are susceptible. And as you age, you become more prone to it. Metabolic syndrome is the early warning system for far more serious problems. If you suffer from several of the above conditions, you are at great risk for future heart problems, stroke, cognitive decline, a vastly weakened immune system, and a long list of potentially fatal illnesses that are all rooted in inactivity (Futurity 2016).

## Obesity Reaches Epidemic Levels

According to the World Health Organization (WHO), about 13 percent of adults worldwide are obese (*Medical News Today* 2019). In the United States, the situation is even more concerning, with almost 40 percent of the adult population living with this condition.

If you require another reason to go for a walk as soon as possible, consider that obesity is linked to smaller brains (Design Fitness Center 2019). In fact, obesity will literally shrink your brain, and that can have serious consequences later in life, including early-onset dementia and possibly Alzheimer's. So really, get up and go for a walk.

## Dementia Risk

As people live longer inactive lives, it's a real risk that their bodies will last longer than their brains. Meaning, we can expect to see many more cases of people living longer but with diminished cognitive abilities. Many are already concerned about this possibility. In surveys, fear of cognitive decline ranks right up there with fear of cancer, and rightly so. It's terrifying to think about losing the essence of who you are yet remaining alive in the shell of your body.

The decline into Alzheimer's is disorienting and dangerous for the person experiencing the transition, but it's also highly stressful for family and friends. Alzheimer's is also one of the most expensive conditions to care for. The lifetime cost of care for a person with dementia is estimated to be $342,000 (Sherry Christiansen 2018).

A recent meta-analysis reported that the global prevalence of dementia is somewhere between five and seven percent in people aged 60 or over. By the age of 85 years and older, between 25 and 50 percent of people display symptoms of dementia and, more specifically, Alzheimer's.

Since the 85 and older group is one of the fastest-growing age groups, and this group is most susceptible to dementia and Alzheimer's, something needs to be done to manage the rapidly growing amount of dementia and Alzheimer's cases.

## Excessive Stress Abounds

The American Institute of Stress reports that in 2018, one-third of US-based respondents visited a doctor for something stress-related. Sixty-three percent of US workers are ready to quit their jobs due to stress, and stress caused sleep deprivation in 66 percent of American workers.

I once took a stress management seminar at work. The presenters advised participants that after the seminar, we were likely to feel more stressed because we were now more aware of all the things in our lives that caused stress (most of them actually seemed to be caused by work). And now that I think about it, isn't it troubling that there actually is a place called the American Institute of Stress?

Stress is a problem not only because of the way it makes you feel but also because of the physiological impact as well. Under great stress, your body produces cortisol. Cortisol is a hormone in your bloodstream that triggers your fight-or-flight response when threatened. Stressful situations can raise your cortisol levels, which makes you more susceptible to weight gain, memory problems, shorter attention span, and even heart problems. It is also thought to inhibit the creation of new brain cells. One thing is certain. You do not want your brain bathed in cortisol on a regular basis.

While it's not possible to eliminate stress from your life entirely (and actually a certain amount of it can be productive), excessive stress is concerning. Being active and getting outside can lessen stress and improve your health.

## A Pill for Everything

Except for the occasional aspirin for headache or pain, I am fortunate because I don't have to take any regular prescriptions. I'm also unusual. Approximately 70 percent of Americans are on some form of medication. That's concerning.

What's more alarming is that, according to the AARP, older Americans are prescribed almost 55 medications per year. That averages out to about four and one-half prescriptions per month. If brand name drugs (not generics) are used to treat chronic conditions, the average annual retail cost for this many medications in 2017 would be approximately $30,591 (Stephen Schondelmeyer 2018).

It's overwhelming that this is what we've come to and that we accept this as normal. I know there's a better way. We have to take control of our personal health, and that means looking beyond prescriptions. Of course, if a medication is needed, it should be taken. But physical health is part of the equation. Doctors should be able to write prescriptions for fitness, walking, and hiking. It would make all of us healthier.

So, that's the bad news. We live in a nation of inactive, sedentary, unfit people, and the rest of the world is not far behind.

I'm not the first to say this (and I hope not to be the last), but fitness is medicine. It can reduce the severity of many diseases and improve overall health. Better yet, it's just plain fun. Getting outdoors is the best medicine available. It is cheap, fast, and effective, and it occurs so far "upstream" that it's the ultimate preventive healthcare solution.

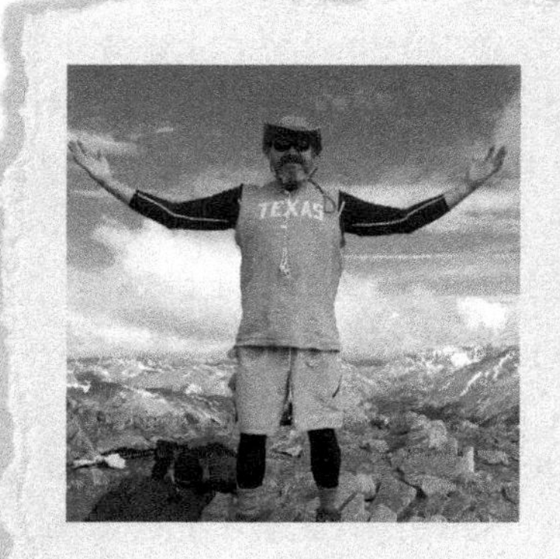


"I was limping from leg surgery and did a lot of flat walking with a loaded pack to work up to walking 20 miles at a time. Showed up in Colorado. Hiked Mt Elbert. It was the hardest thing I'd ever done and, without a doubt, the most satisfying. Since then, I've returned every year and climbed two or three 14ers. I struggle. My right leg still doesn't work right, but I love hiking to the point that I plan to move to Colorado. I'm going to climb as many mountains as I can for as long as I can."

– Kevin Brumfield, Texas

# 7

# WAY, WAY UPSTREAM PREVENTIVE HEALTHCARE

*Fitness for the young person is an option, but for the older person it is an imperative, as frailty and death linger nearby.*

– WALTER BORTZ, MD

The only true preventive healthcare—where prevention is defined as "the action of stopping something from happening"—occurs long before you show symptoms. It occurs before you need the medical and pharma system and long before you go to the doctor with a problem. It happens every day as you decide how you live your life, the choices you make, what you eat, and especially how you approach fitness.

Unfortunately, Big Medicine and Big Pharma are not focused enough on actual prevention or actual cures. Rather, they seem focused on providing continuous, expensive, and profitable treatments that address symptoms but often fail to solve the primary problem. I don't consider that prevention.

We have amazing new medical and pharmacological innovations, unimaginable only a generation ago, that can extend life and stall once-fatal diseases. But at the same time, we are all concerned about the increasingly high cost, availability, and limitations of healthcare, and increasingly skeptical of a medical and pharmacological business model that often views us not as patients, but as long-term, living, recurring revenue streams.

Get someone on blood pressure or anti-cholesterol meds at age 40, and they can be customers for 30, 40, or 50 years, paid for by insurance. Where's the incentive to cure cancer or Alzheimer's when it's more profitable just to slow, manage, and prolong it for ten, fifteen, or more years?

Where's the incentive to prevent disease from happening in the first place? And why do we spend so much money on healthcare when nature has so much 'free medicine' to offer?

The real solution to the healthcare crisis is a focus on actual prevention, or rather what some people are starting to call "upstream preventive healthcare." It occurs so far upstream that the problem never exists. Cure metabolic syndrome, diabetes, and high blood pressure by staying lean and fit, thus preventing obesity from ever occurring. Cure heart disease by keeping your heart muscle strong and preventing your vascular system from clogging up. Cure sarcopenia and osteoporosis by preventing muscles and bones from getting weak and frail in the first place.

Who makes money on upstream prevention? Well, you do actually. If you prevent yourself from getting sick, getting obese, or developing any aspect of metabolic syndrome, you spend less on medical care. So, you have more money. Simple. The best way to get this far upstream is fitness, and the best way to get the maximum benefit of this fitness is to do it outside.

## Very Troubling Statistics

Chronic diseases and the health risk behaviors that cause them account for the majority of healthcare costs. Since these are mostly the result of lifestyle choices, they are often quite preventable. And while genetics, diet, and environment also play a role in these preventable diseases, lifestyle choice and the amount of exercise you get are key factors that can reduce their likelihood.

### Annual Deaths by Type

| # | *USA* | *(000's)* | *Global* | *(millions)* |
|---|---|---|---|---|
| *1.* | Heart disease | 635 | Heart disease | 9.3 |
| *2.* | Cancer | 598 | Stroke | 5.9 |
| 3. | Accidents | 161 | Pulmonary disease | 3 |
| *4.* | Respiratory diseases | 154 | Respiratory diseases | 3 |
| *5.* | Stroke | 142 | Alzheimer's | 2.1 |
| *6.* | Alzheimer's | 116 | Lung disease | 2 |
| *7.* | Diabetes | 80 | Diabetes | 1.9 |
| *8.* | Flu / Pneumonia | 51 | Road injury | 1.8 |
| *9.* | Kidney disease | 50 | Diarrheal diseases | 1.6 |
| *10.* | Suicide | 45 | Tuberculosis | 1.4 |

*(Center For Disease Control and Prevention 2020)*

Here's the problem: prevention doesn't sell, and it isn't as profitable for the healthcare ecosystem. (However, investing in the kind of prevention that fitness creates would be profitable for the health insurance industry). The human psyche seems to always be in denial that something bad can happen to them … until it happens. Then, we try to reverse and undo it. For some reason, and against all logic, most people make a few bad lifestyle choices (some make a lot of them) that contribute directly to their own significant and expensive illnesses, disease, and death.

Only when a health problem surfaces, and there are symptoms to react to, do we try to fix it. By then, we're not really preventing anything. We're merely trying to keep it from getting worse—pre-diabetes, pre-heart disease, pre-dementia. If you're in the "pre" phase, it is not really prevention. It's the early stage of something that probably could have been avoided completely if you were practicing real upstream preventive healthcare (i.e., living a fitness lifestyle).

---

*"Those who think they have not time for bodily exercise will sooner or later have to find time for illness."*

**– Edward Stanley**

---

## What Enhanced Fitness Prevents

Fitness has benefits for every cell in your body. It works as a preventive measure, it works as a treatment to cure illness, and it helps you recover faster should you get sick. The fitter you are, the quicker you recover from surgery and medical procedures. More specifically, consider these examples:

## Heart Disease

The fitter you are, the less likely you are to suffer from any kind of heart disease. Being fit strengthens the heart muscle and significantly reduces the chance of cardiovascular illnesses, like heart attacks, clogged arteries (atherosclerosis), or hardening of the arteries (arteriosclerosis). A strong heart muscle also improves circulation to your entire body, and that benefits all of your bodily organs and processes.

## Hypertension

High blood pressure is part of the metabolic syndrome cluster of symptoms. Untreated high blood pressure can lead to stroke, heart attack, kidney disease, early dementia, and is most often treated with a program of long-term medication. In many of these cases (specifically the ones not associated with a genetic component), regular physical activity can prevent, reduce, and control high blood pressure.

## Cancer

In a landmark 2016 study, the American Cancer Society and the National Cancer Institute researchers found that exercise was associated with a significantly decreased risk of colon cancer, breast cancer, endometrial cancer, esophageal cancer, liver cancer, stomach cancer, kidney cancer, and myeloid leukemia. The study found this was due in part because it helps with weight management; however, it was also found to help better regulate hormones, insulin levels, and the immune system. Physical activity was found to be "strongly associated with a decreased risk of multiple myeloma, a blood cancer, as well as cancers of the head and neck, rectum, bladder, and lung (in current and former smokers)" (American Cancer Society 2016).

The Mayo Clinic even goes so far as to call exercise a secret weapon and one of the most important elements of cancer treatment. Sara Mansfield, M.S., a certified cancer exercise trainer with the Mayo Clinic Healthy Living Program, says, "Physical activity can help people before, during, and after cancer treatment. Research tells us, in general, it's better to move more than less" (Mayo Clinic 2019).

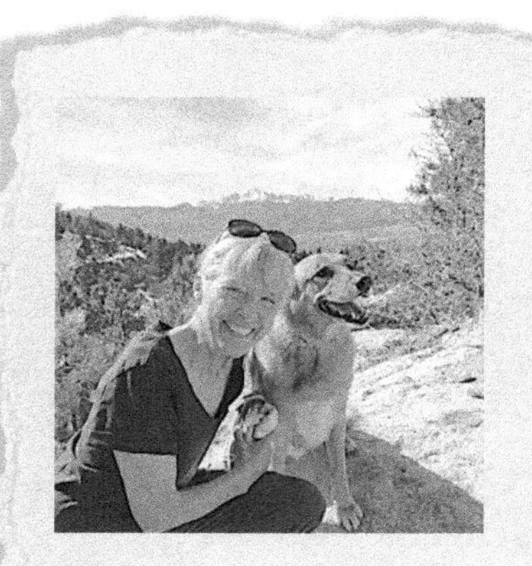

"When I climbed the highest mountain in Colorado, I still had drainage tubes coming out of my side after my mastectomy two weeks earlier. Doing that climb gave me the certainty that I was still me, and nothing else could have accomplished that. Many years later, I broke my back, and I turned to the same source of healing. And by healing, I mean all of me—mind, body and spirit. Now 75, I've found over and over that as soon as I get outside, breathe in the fresh air, and get my body moving, I instantly feel better! It's the synergy of putting it all together that is magical for me."

– Susan Mitchell, Colorado

## Diabetes

Diabetes is a disease where your body's ability to produce or respond to insulin is weakened. Insulin is a hormone that regulates blood glucose (sugar), which is a source of energy for the body. This weakening causes an abnormal metabolizing of carbohydrates and elevated levels of glucose in the blood and urine. Type 2 diabetes is one of the metabolic syndrome factors, and its symptoms include frequent urination, increased thirst and hunger, fatigue, and numbness in hands and feet. Obesity is believed to account for 80 to 85 percent of the risk of developing type 2 diabetes. Research suggests that an obese person is up to 80 times more likely to develop type 2 diabetes than those with a lean body type (*Diabetes and Obesity* 2019).

## Flu / Pneumonia

Viral respiratory infections represent the most common form of infectious disease and account for over seven percent of all deaths. Deaths associated with respiratory viral infections occur most often in the elderly and other immune-compromised individuals whose immune systems are incapable of handling an elevated viral load. Researchers have found that "prolonged, intense exercise causes immunosuppression, while moderate-intensity exercise improves immune function and potentially reduces risk and severity of respiratory viral infection." Based on available evidence, moderate-intensity exercise training should be used as an adjunct to other preventive measures against respiratory tract viral infection (Martin 2009).

## Sarcopenia

This condition is the gradual loss of muscle, including mass, strength, size, quality/elasticity, power, and stamina. It typically begins during your forties. Simply put, it is the weakness we associate with aging and largely the result of age plus inactivity. It happens so gradually it's hard to notice until, all of a sudden, you're frail. Your muscles have shriveled, and your bones are unprotected and brittle.

The good news is that the onset of sarcopenia can be delayed for many years, and it is a somewhat reversible condition. Resistance training and weight-bearing exercises are essential to prevent or slow its onset. With proper exercise, it is even possible to reverse it. According to Nathan LeBrasseur of the Mayo Clinic in Rochester, Minnesota, exercise is "Without question ... the most powerful intervention to address muscle loss, whether it occurs in the context of advancing age or debilitating chronic or acute diseases" (Mayo Clinic 2014).

So, our fitness goals should include a bonus of providing us with upstream preventive healthcare. It's occurring so far upstream that you cannot see or hear the waterfalls or rapids—before you have chest pains, before you have symptoms like shortness of breath, or before you have an expanded waistline.

Some doctors are finally getting it, but far too few. Many continue to treat conditions and plan to wait until long-term, evidence-based research and peer-reviewed studies support upstream preventive measures. I believe it's time to begin the transition. Doctors need to add prescriptions for fitness to their treatment plans.

## Fall Prevention

I want to highlight something most people wouldn't think about as being preventive health care, but since we are addressing the idea of prevention, we need to go way upstream and talk about fall prevention.

Did you know that falls are the leading cause of accidental death in the senior population? One in four seniors falls every year—broken wrists, broken arms, and the dreaded broken hip. Two and one-half million seniors per year are treated for these injuries, and it costs over $60 billion dollars in yearly healthcare costs.

Well, the fitness you will attain through walking, hiking, and the related functional fitness exercises we recommend, in a very direct way, is the best way to prevent falls and their expensive consequences. This kind of fitness gives you the balance to prevent falls from happening in the first place. It gives you the quick reflexes and muscle speed you need to recover from trips and occasional slips, so instead of falling on your wrist or your hip, you catch yourself before you fall. And the fitter you are, the more flexible you are, the stronger your bones, the denser your muscles, and so it is more likely that if you do fall, you won't be injured.

Personally, I'm an expert at this. I've taken a few spectacular falls recently—went through the handlebars of my bike to avoid a darting dog onto a bike trail, tripped headfirst over a tree root while descending a steep trail in New Hampshire, and even slipped on the ice running in my driveway. I've survived these falls with only minor bumps and bruises. I'm certain a less fit person, or frailer person, would not be so lucky. Fall prevention is perhaps one of the least recognized elements of preventive health care. Because these statistics

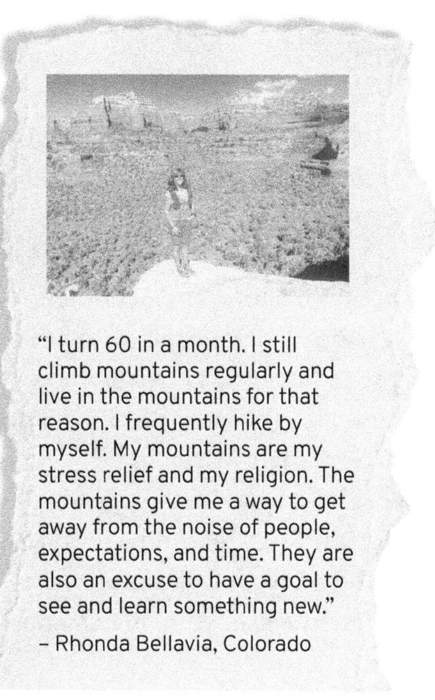

"I turn 60 in a month. I still climb mountains regularly and live in the mountains for that reason. I frequently hike by myself. My mountains are my stress relief and my religion. The mountains give me a way to get away from the noise of people, expectations, and time. They are also an excuse to have a goal to see and learn something new."

– Rhonda Bellavia, Colorado

are practically impossible to track, it's hard to demonstrate, but fall prevention can and does save lives, and it significantly reduces healthcare costs.

## The Uphill Cure

The more time you spend outdoors, the healthier you will be. The more time you spend walking uphill, the more benefits you will accrue for your brain and body.

Living close to nature and spending time outside has significant and wide-ranging health benefits. A new report from the University of East Anglia reveals that exposure to greenspace reduces the risk of type 2 diabetes, cardiovascular disease, premature death, preterm birth, stress, and high blood pressure. Researchers found that people who lived near greenspaces benefited in two ways. They had more options for socializing and physical activity, and they were exposed to "a diverse variety of bacteria present in natural areas," which may enhance their immune system and decrease inflammation (University of East Anglia 2018).

Big Healthcare and Big Pharma make a lot less money if you are fit and healthy. Their business models depend on a never-ending stream of sick people who need tests, doctor visits, prescriptions, procedures, surgeries, and so on. All of these services are often ridiculously overpriced and padded. It amounts to trillions of dollars each year.

So, stay active and get fit. You will be amazed by how medically boring your life can be and how much more satisfying it is NOT to be a revenue stream for the medical community. If you don't want to waste your life savings and your retirement income on doctors, pills, and massive medical expenses, being fit and active gives you the best chance.

---

*"We do not stop exercising because we grow old – we grow old because we stop exercising."*

**– Dr. Kenneth Cooper**

---

# 8
# FITNESS IS MEDICINE

*If this were a drug, we would be giving it to all our patients.*

– Kaitlin Casaletto, Ph.D., assistant professor of neurology, UCSF

If things are pretty good for you already, being fit makes it only go better. If things aren't going so well, being fit can give you the willpower, the energy, and the confidence to turn it around. Being fit allows you to access your full potential, to unleash the best version of yourself, and to experience more fully every aspect of your life.

Being fit is not just about recreational activities and playing sports. Being fit permits you to function more effectively in the world: lift a suitcase, shovel snow, rearrange the furniture, carry a box of books up the stairs, walk the dog, drive your car more safely, and so on.

And being fit keeps you independent. If you want to work, you can. If you want to travel, you can. If you want to walk across Spain on the Camino de Santiago Trail or hike sections of the Appalachian Trail, you can. Heck, how about this: if you want to go for a walk in the park with your great-grandchildren, you can.

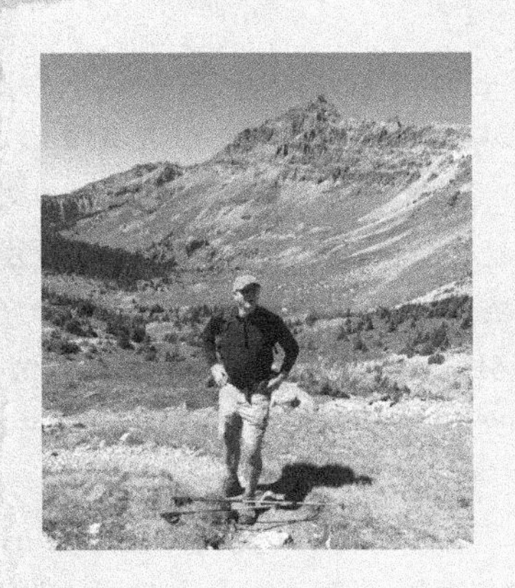

"I am a retired pilot and feel hiking is like flying. You are continually managing the risks. As we get older, the risks change, the pace gets slower, but the peaks can still be had. The best physical conditioning I know is to put a pack on your back and go hiking."

– Ray Wild, Colorado

If you don't want to exhaust your life savings and your retirement benefits on medical expenses, if you don't want to spend the last ten years of your life drugged up and being driven from one doctor's office to another, being fit and active now gives you the best chance.

Here are some of the benefits of fitness:

## 1. Fitness Gives Your Immune System a Boost

A stronger immune system is a fitness bonus supported by numerous studies. One investigation found that even moderate exercise appears to have a "beneficial effect on the immune function, which could protect against upper respiratory tract infections" (Jeurissen 2003).

The benefits of fitness are especially helpful as you get older since your immune system goes into a decline as you age. The more you exercise, the more blood and oxygen courses through your body, and that creates a powerful anti-inflammatory effect.

Exercising and spending time outdoors provide an extra boost. Vitamin D strengthens the immune system, so time spent outside in the sun is time well spent. Additionally, being exposed to the sun helps your body to convert cholesterol into vitamin D.

The final immune boost from fitness is that it makes your body stronger and better able to fight off cold, flu, and other illnesses.

Professor Knut Wittkowski, head of Rockefeller University's Department of Biostatistics, Epidemiology, and Research Design, would agree: "The flu ends during springtime when people spend more time outdoors because in the outdoors viruses cannot easily spread. Going outdoors is what stops every respiratory disease" (Wittkowsk 2020).

## 2. Fit People Are Healthier in General

The more frequently you exercise, and the more intense that exercise is, the greater the health benefits. Hiking can be about as intense as it gets. Intense exercise also significantly reduces the likelihood of cancer, diabetes, dementia, stroke, and cardiovascular disease. Fit people who do weight-bearing exercise—and hiking is weight-bearing—build stronger bones, making them more resistant to falls and other accidents (Ballantyne 2009).

## 3. Fit People Live Longer

Now there is science-based evidence that as little as 15 minutes of vigorous exercise each day can have tremendous longevity benefits. There is also clear statistical proof that not exercising at all significantly increases your risk of early death. More compelling is the research being done on the older population. The Human Performance Laboratory at Ball State University discovered that "people in their 70s who exercise regularly can have the heart, lung, and muscle fitness of healthy people 30 years younger" (Crouch 2019).

Another report in the *British Journal of Sports Medicine* indicates that exercise can be spaced out throughout a full day and even ten minutes of vigorous exercise here and there have a clear impact on lifespan (Sifferlin 2018). So just think about this for a second and realize how easy it would be to add two or three 10-minute bursts of physical activity to your day.

## 4. Fit People Have Bigger Brains

The average human brain after the age of 40 naturally begins to shrink, typically by about five percent per year. However, people who maintain a high degree of fitness are able to drastically slow and reverse the deterioration. Being fit has great benefits for your brain (NICM 2017).

Conversely, an obese person's brain can be up to eight percent smaller than a fit person's. Research at the Cleveland Clinic looked at people with an average age of 55 and found that a high percentage of body fat is linked to having a smaller brain (Cleveland Clinic Newsroom 2019). Being sedentary and obese can literally shrink your brain.

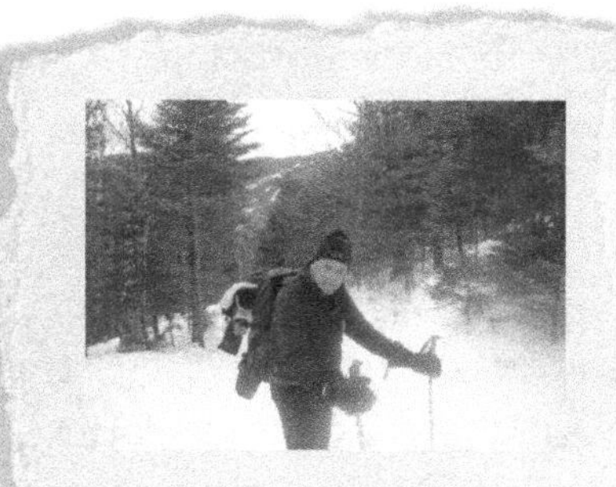

"I am almost 81. I have been hiking for 21 years. In 1980, I had a triple bypass. In 1996, I had a quadruple bypass, and about nine years ago, I had my left knee replaced. For the last four to five years, I haven't had to have a stress test because my cardiologist said my hiking and going to the gym was my stress test, so apparently my body grew some veins and small arteries, and so I haven't had any chest pain for that length of time, and I attribute that to going to the gym and hiking. Went hiking yesterday, my Fitbit read 17,000 steps, 7.81 miles, 77 floors, not too shabby for 81!"

– Allan Hewitt, Maine

### 5. It's Never Too Late to Start

Studies now show unfit people as old as age 79 who have never exercised can receive significant benefits by increasing activity level and beginning an exercise program. Inactive people at that age decreased their mortality rate by 24 percent due to an increase in physical activity. "There are clearly benefits at all levels" of activity, said lead researcher Soren Brage, a principal investigator with the MRC Epidemiology Unit at the University of Cambridge. "The most encouraging is you don't have to be a super-athlete, and it's never too late" (Lemar 2019).

## Live Long, Die Fast

The worst-case, end-of-life scenario is a long, slow, complicated, painful, and expensive decline. The attainable goal, and a much better alternative, is a long, active, healthy life, and then a rapid decline to morbidity. This can be made much more feasible by practicing a fitness-is-medicine lifestyle.

The fact is you can take charge of the way you age by choosing to be fit. That choice can change the trajectory of your aging. You do not have to go on a long, slow, medically expensive decline into inactivity, illness, and dependency. You want to live longer, live life to the fullest, see your great-grandchildren, be more productive, and have more fun, right? Well, your chances go way up if you choose to be fit. The term for this is compressed morbidity. It is the only way to go.

I recently saw 13 wheelchairs lined up at a single airline departure gate. The average age of these folks? Fifties and sixties. No broken legs, no obvious injuries. Just a group of unfit, obese, and morbidly obese people who were not able to walk the 1,000 steps to the airport gate while rolling a light carry-on bag. Too large and unfit to walk across the airport, they each needed an aide to push them and help them onto the plane.

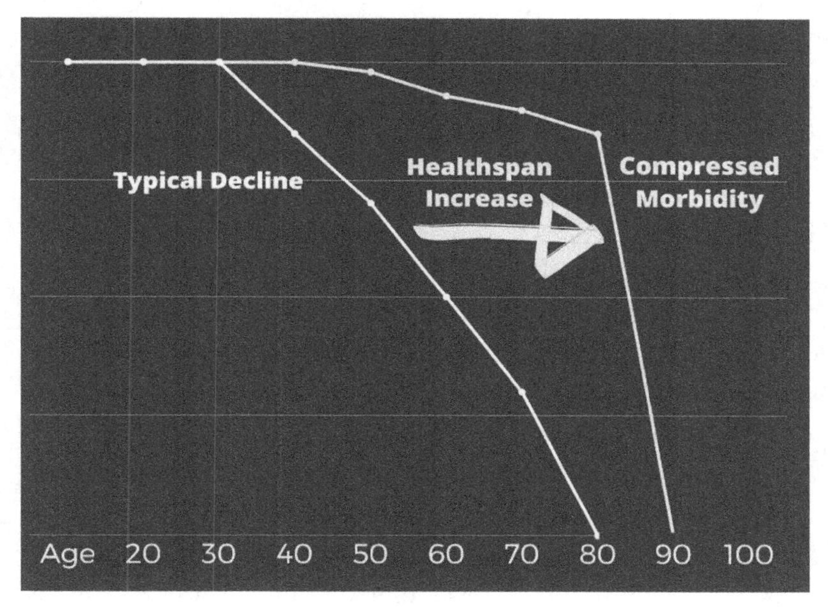


*Typical Trajectory of Aging v. Compressed Morbidity*

How did it ever come to this? How sad for those 13 people. What a burden this is—for the families of these people, for society, and for the airline.

I didn't have to see any medical records to know that I was looking at 13 cases of advanced metabolic syndrome. There surely was heart disease, diabetes, high blood pressure, and obesity, not to mention ankle, knee, and hip problems from years of carrying that extra weight around and being sedentary.

Thirteen cases of people whose lifestyle and behavioral choices were likely going to shorten their lives. But before that happens, I see medical bills, perpetual prescriptions, continuous doctor and hospital expenses, and the misery of a constrained and unproductive life.

I see numerous angioplasties for $15,000 each. High blood pressure and hypertension medication at $1,000 and up per year. I see joint replacements at $50,000 per knee or $40,000 per hip. I see heart valve surgeries at $60,000 each. I see pacemaker implantations at $40,000 each. You get the picture. That's just a short list of the possibilities that will befall those 13 people. And at a population level, as the older population increases, the cost of this is staggering.

These people are going to die from self-inflicted wounds. It's not suicide, but it is, to some extent, a choice. It didn't have to be this way. Better lifestyle choices and more time spent on fitness could have prevented this.

So now you see that fitness is not only medicine, it's actually much more than that. Fitness is upstream preventive healthcare. It occurs so far upstream that, at a population level, it significantly reduces the need for medical intervention, drugs, and many healthcare services. Fitness can be one of the most important parts of the long-term healthcare equation.

# 9

# UNPLUG TO FIND THE JOBO

*Do not even listen, simply wait, be quiet, still and solitary. The world will freely offer itself to you to be unmasked, it has no choice, it will roll in ecstasy at your feet.*

— FRANZ KAFKA

Instead of the world rolling in ecstasy at my feet, as I was writing this chapter, the world sent me 21 text messages, four LinkedIn pings, 16 Facebook alerts, 35 Instagram alerts, eight phone calls, 65 emails (35 of them junk), a weather alert, two WhatsApp messages, two Fitbit pings, one squirrel set off the backyard motion detector six times, and I was added to a Messenger thread with 20 people that pinged my phone 40 times in one hour. That surely can get in the way of any ecstasy the world had intended for me.

We live in strange times. Marvelous new technology everywhere, but instead of looking up and off to the horizon for inspiration, we look down and at a little screen for too many hours. Instead of getting out there and seeing the world, we can live vicariously through others posting their own adventures on YouTube, Facebook, and Instagram.

If you're reading this, you almost certainly have a smartphone, a tablet, a computer, and social media or email accounts. You have succumbed to the lure of digital connectivity. It's become hard to live and work without these tools: they are nearly irresistible, very addictive, and endlessly distracting.

The same nearly inconceivable situation exists at Mount Everest. On the entire 50-mile route through Nepal from Lukla Airport to the mountain, there is a cell signal and internet connectivity nearly every step of the way. On a recent trek in, my whole team, myself included, was continuously preoccupied with Instagram posting, messages to family and friends a world away, and checking email. At both breakfast and dinner, rather than absorbing the spectacle of where we were and what we were about to accomplish that day, almost everyone was posting, texting, and talking with people in Australia, South Africa, the UK, and the USA.

I did it as well. I wanted to chronicle where I was, what I was doing, share some of the experience with friends back home, and reassure family that I was still alive. The GPS device I carried was beaming my precise location up to a satellite and onto a webpage in real time. While I applaud its ability to make my adventures safer and marvel at the technology, it's also just one more device that pulls me away from being present in the moment.

I even checked the security system cameras at home, for no other reason than because I could. It was surreal to see my car parked in the driveway back home in Connecticut, in real time on my phone, while I was sitting in a tea house in Gorak Shep, Nepal, at 17,000 feet above sea level and 100 miles from the nearest road. One of my trek mates was constantly checking the status of his Tesla sitting at home in Colorado, and he even started it up a few times for us to see.

This is not what I was expecting in remote and rugged Nepal. Reliable digital connectivity on virtually every step of the trail. Sherpa porters, whose job it is to ferry supplies up and down the route, are now killing time while laden with gargantuan loads by talking on the phone, texting, taking selfies, and Facebooking. Instead of the polite traditional greeting of 'namaste,' most of the porters you cross paths with zoom right past you while conversing with someone far away.

All of these digital distractions make me wonder if digital tools, most well-meaning and merely trying to make our lives easier or more efficient and productive, have, in some ways, made us less productive. I think we are so susceptible to the individual logic of each one of these tools that we have missed the bigger point—having so many digital gadgets shouting for our attention, in many ways, makes us less efficient.

Truth be told, no one is immune to the lure of digital distractions, and they are here to stay. Going forward, the real challenge will be to manage these constant distractions. We need to carve out time to unplug, and that will take vigilance and discipline.

This is harder than it sounds. Research has shown that "social media cues, such as 'likes' on one of our posts or pictures, trigger a surge in dopamine, the neurotransmitter associated with pleasure and reward, which may diminish the motivation to pay attention to anything else" (Haynes 2020). That's pretty powerful and difficult to manage.

With all these alerts crying for attention (a beep, a chime, a ring, a song) and each one trying to stand out to give you information, the net effect is that you're going to learn to shut them out. You eventually train your brain to ignore the alerts intended to help you be more productive, even the really important ones. But you can't really ignore them.

All of these notifications become a sea of static. While you can push the static into the background, your brain still hears it all. It has to expend extra energy to filter out these signals, and the result is you're expending extra energy to ignore things, which makes your brain tired. If you're still connected and filtering out alerts, warnings, and beeps, you're not really unplugged, and you're not resting your brain.

I am somewhat of an expert on this plugged versus unplugged tug of war. I like many aspects of digital technology, so I've tended to be an early adopter, and I'm very susceptible to the lure of it all. I'm as wired as any millennial, and I'm hands-on with social media for some of my companies. I'm constantly connected with two smartphones and a bunch of computers that keep me busy with texts, 300 emails a day from multiple time zones, and countless notifications.

I once held a job where people peppered me from all around the world, and where work was done 24/7. This means I could log on at 2 am at home and be in a real-time chat with someone in Australia, Hong Kong, India, or South Africa. It's very easy to get pulled into thinking that the more you do, the more productive you are. You start to think the world will stop spinning if you don't instantly respond, merely because you can. In truth, I do like being "plugged in" to things and people all over the world. But you have to draw the line somewhere; your brain can't be switched on 24/7, 365 days a year.

Here's what I've learned: if you don't unplug and disconnect regularly, if you don't shut everything off, your brain included, said brain gets tired. It gets distracted, and you become less creative, less effective, and less present, even though you're spending more hours doing things.

Even your eyesight becomes strained, and your vision narrows because you're focusing all your attention on a tiny screen and tiny print right in front of your face. We didn't evolve for this.

Our brains like us to be moving and for our scope of vision to be broad, looking for predators and dangers (like charging lions or speeding cars) in order to stay properly stimulated and exercised. We've already learned that sitting is the enemy of fitness. Well, staring at a screen is a big part of why we are sitting so much.

So, from time to time, we badly need a digital detox.

And, heck, if you can't unplug, try to slow down. Must everything be instantaneous? I don't think our brains can completely handle all this technology, speed, and excessive information. Just because you can be connected 24/7 does not mean it is necessarily a good thing.

Staring at screens all day and then watching television at night creates a narrow mind. I think it's not good to spend so much time in a two-dimensional world. It's flat; it doesn't move. It lacks so much of what makes a complete sensory experience.

If you get outside and unplug, you gain a full, three-dimensional experience. It has depth. It has the richness and expansiveness that is so lacking when you're indoors staring at screens.

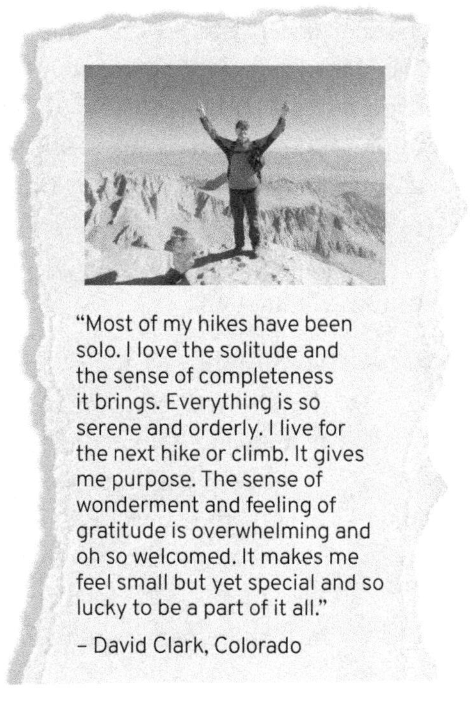

"Most of my hikes have been solo. I love the solitude and the sense of completeness it brings. Everything is so serene and orderly. I live for the next hike or climb. It gives me purpose. The sense of wonderment and feeling of gratitude is overwhelming and oh so welcomed. It makes me feel small but yet special and so lucky to be a part of it all."

– David Clark, Colorado

So, it's important to schedule in time at least once a week when you turn everything off. It gives you a chance to relax and recharge.

Unplug from technology as often as possible. Staring at a computer monitor plus your phone's ringing, pinging, and dinging randomly all day and sometimes all night is a real detriment not only to your attention span but also to your brain health and stress levels. Shut off all but the most important alerts, unplug totally at night and retrain yourself to enjoy the silence.

## Forget FOMO ... Seek JOBO

I know you've heard of FOMO. It's the fear of missing out. It's that little twinge of anxiety you get from seeing your Facebook and Instagram 'friends' posting about their fabulous jet-set doings, luxury meals, and so on, and realizing you're not as fabulous. Well, forget it. Ignore FOMO, unplug from time to time, and experience JOBO—the joy of being outside. It forces you to unplug and reframe your thinking to experience what's directly around you. You get more joy for yourself and discover the joy of missing out.

What you will find if you do this regularly is that several things will happen:

1. Your ability to focus on the present will be improved, thereby reducing much of the attention deficit disorder that always being connected fosters.
2. Your sleep will improve. Forty-four percent of us actually sleep with our phones, so we don't miss anything. This is up from, say, zero percent before smartphones.
3. You might actually have more conversations with live human beings, in person.

Here's something else to try: no music on your run, workout, or hike. Many of you think that pounding, high-decibel music is a motivator for a good workout. There are articles and recommendations everywhere about the best playlists to blast into your earphones while working out, walking, jogging, or running. I have my favorite playlists too, but I've increasingly been opting for silence and take that active time to spend listening to the natural world.

For many, and this is little known or understood, high-impact music creates unwanted stress and tension that triggers the creation of the stress hormone, cortisol, which, in excess amounts, leads to weight gain, anxiety, depression, and worst of all, can harm brain cells. So, turn the volume way down or turn it off and listen to the quiet.

## Mindfulness

There has been a lot of discussion in the last decade about mindfulness as people look for relief from the stressful, digital lives we lead. If you're not familiar with the concept, mindfulness is "the psychological process of purposely bringing one's attention to experiences occurring in the present moment without judgment, which one can develop through the practice of meditation and through other training." It is also considered "a mental state achieved by focusing one's awareness on the present moment, while calmly acknowledging and accepting one's feelings, thoughts, and bodily sensations, used as a therapeutic technique" (Wikipedia 2020).

There is a staggering number of seminars, webinars, classes, experts, and apps to teach you mindfulness. Critics of mindfulness make the case that it is overhyped, a placebo, or snake oil, largely because it is now big business for some practitioners. I think mindfulness is a critical part of the stress management equation, and I have tried numerous options in this arena. I suggest trying a few to see what works for you.

---

*"To spend a lengthy period alone in the forests or mountains, a period of coming to terms with the solitude and nonhumanity of nature is to discover who, or what, one really is—a discovery hardly possible while the community is telling you what you are or ought to be."*

**– Alan Watts**

---

## Be Present

The goal of mindfulness is to focus on the present moment. This keeps your mind attentive to what's around you, and as a result, stress levels naturally decrease, sleep improves, and creativity climbs. I've found the best way for me to focus on the present moment and to find my version of mindfulness is to unplug and go for a hike—the harder, the better.

Many researchers and doctors agree with me. The act of going outside and walking in nature connects us to the world, ourselves, and those around us. The quiet of the trees, the sounds of birds, and the physical act of walking or hiking focuses your mind on the world around you and fosters mental and physical rejuvenation.

For those of you who want to gain these benefits but are taking your first steps, consider beginning with the practice of forest bathing, which simply means going outside into nature and moving. Some trace this practice back to Japan, where it is known as shinrin-yoku, or taking in the forest. The beauty of this practice is that you can experience it in the forest, a nearby park, at the beach, along a river, or any number of outdoor locations.

While free and easily accessible, forest bathing is also now available as the focal point of high-end vacations. Luxury hotels and spas, like the Mohonk Mountain House in New Paltz, New York, promote it as an opportunity for "mindfulness and recreation and renewal of body, mind, and spirit in a beautiful natural setting." They offer walks complete with a one-on-one session with a mindfulness coach (Mohonk Mountain House 2020).

For people who have struggled unsuccessfully with meditation and mindfulness techniques, my hunch is that this will work better.

My version of mindfulness, as you might expect, is solo hiking and climbing. According to *Psychology Today*, mindfulness is "a state of

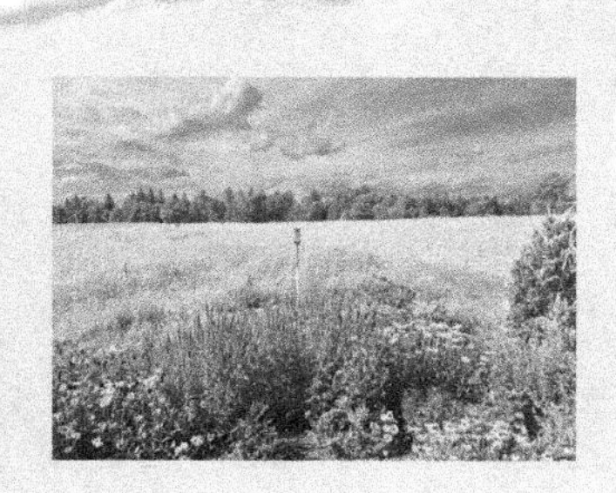

*Topsmeade State Forest, Connecticut*

Two hours a week outside can change your life. A long walk outdoors helps keep your serotonin levels up. This helps raise your energy and keeps your mood calm, positive, and focused. Studies show that it's not just the activity. It's the "greenness" of the outdoor space (White 2019).

active, open attention to the present" (Mindfulness 2020). When I'm hiking across a mountain ridge with a 200-foot drop-off to my left and a 1,000-foot slope-off into the wilderness to my right, the exertion and focus required to be safe and in the moment is precisely the state of "attention to the present" mindfulness trainers talk about. Heightened sensory inputs from all sides, especially at altitude where I'm breathing heavily and straining upwards, combined with the possibility of injury if I trip is the best mindfulness there is.

A 20- or 30-minute guided session with a mindfulness app or coach provides great benefits. But a day-long hike is exponentially better, and the results last longer. Imagine what two or three consecutive days on the trail can do for your state of mind.

My solution to unplugging from the digital world is to find a high place—a mountain, a hill, or even a tall building. If you cannot get to the top of something, try a beach, along a river, or even near a wide field. From your selected vantage point, look to the horizon. Look at a broad vista and feel the mental boost of the view and space. As you look into the distance, you're using the full range of your eye muscles. Those muscles relax when they are focused to infinity, and your stress level plummets.

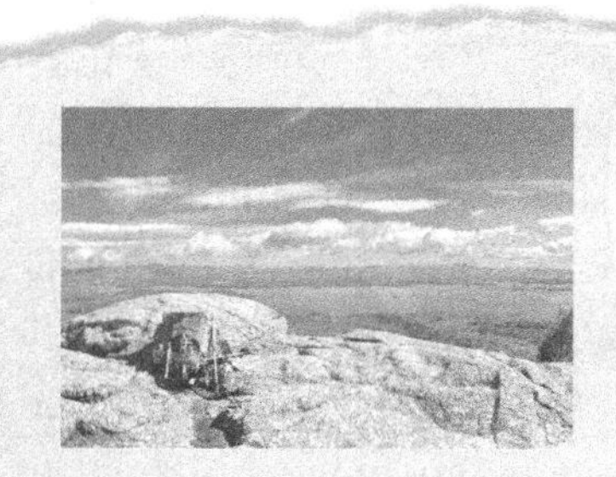

*Mount Major, New Hampshire*

A vista like this can change your perspective on the world, open your mind to new possibilities, and recharge your brain. This amazing overlook on Mount Major in New Hampshire is only an hour from the parking lot yet is a world away from the daily grind. A program of walking, exercise, and hiking can make these places accessible to you.

*"Being connected to everything has disconnected us from ourselves and the preciousness of this present moment."*

– **L.M. Browning**, Vagabonds and Sundries

# THE VIEW FROM ABOVE

I've taken over 100,000,000 uphill steps hiking and climbing on seven continents over 50 years. These steps have helped me discover more about the world and myself than anything else I've done. From the challenges of Antarctica, Everest, and across many of the great mountain ranges of the world to the countless familiar hikes across the hills of the Northeast USA (and especially in New Hampshire's White Mountains), I have found myself.

Somewhere along the way, it hit me that Ansel Adams was spot on when he said: "You are not in the mountains, the mountains are in you." They've been my teacher, my church, my inspiration, and the core of a pretty amazing fitness program for all these years.

That's why I've written this book. I want to share my experience to help others find longer, happier, healthier lives.

I want you to find your own path as you learn some of the secrets of aging well—outside.

## Harpers Ferry, West Virginia

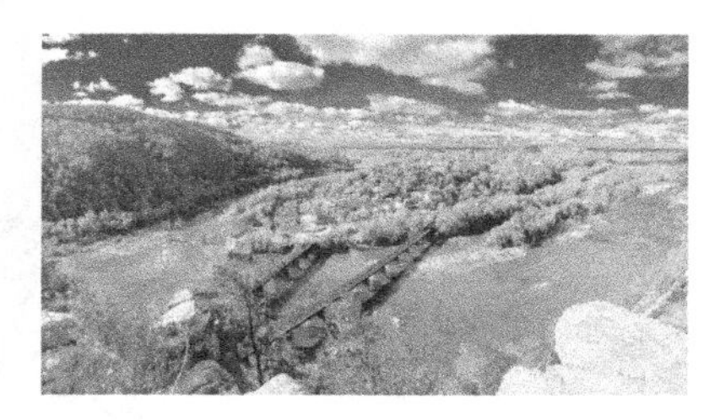

This is the halfway point of the fabled Appalachian Trail, viewed from the Maryland Heights overlook. Located only one hour from the Washington

Monument, you'd be amazed by how accessible the wilderness can be. Beautiful vistas like this are within easy reach of Manhattan, Los Angeles, Las Vegas, and virtually all dense urban areas. Put this into a search engine: "hikes near me," and you're off. See Chapter 16.

## Kancamagus Highway, New Hampshire

I don't mind hiking in the rain. With proper gear, you can safely get outside in wet weather. In fact, bad weather often has big rewards.

One of the most memorable and intense moments in my 50 years of hiking was a driving, torrential thunderstorm followed by pelting hail. An overwhelming sensory experience that was shortly followed by the biggest and most persistent rainbow I've ever witnessed. Surprises like this await as you venture into the hills. See Chapter 16.

## A Brain Workout

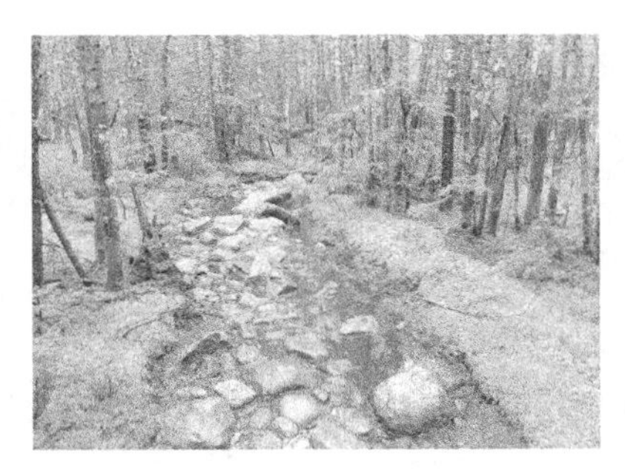

You see a rough and rocky trail. I see a marvelous opportunity to build fitness and brain health. An uneven trail like this requires your eyes, brain, and body to work together in concert. With every step, you must coordinate movements, foot and leg positioning, and balance. As you adapt to the terrain, you also have an elevated heart rate from the exertion. These are the ingredients for building a sharper brain that is more resistant to cognitive decline. Cognitive load plus physical exertion is called dual tasking, and it is very good for your brain. See Chapter 13.

## Forest Bathing

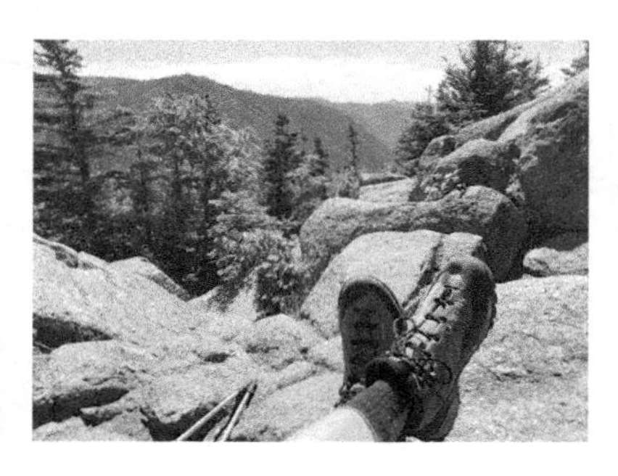

For people who have struggled unsuccessfully with meditation and mindfulness techniques, my hunch is that hiking will work better. My solution to unplugging from the digital world is to find a high place in the sun and look out at a broad vista. You'll start to feel a mental boost from the view and space. Not only will your stress level plummet, but the sunshine provides extra vitamin D. This gives a boost to your immune system, making you more resistant to illness. The natural world contains huge doses of preventive medicine for both brain and body. See Chapters 7 and 9.

## Perspective from Monta Rosa, above Zermatt, Switzerland

"You cannot stay on the summit forever. You have to come down again. So, what's the point? Only this: what is above knows what is below, what is below does not know what is above …

"There is an art to finding your way in the lower regions by the memory of what you have seen when you were higher up. When you can no longer see, you can at least still know." Mount Analogue, Rene Daumal

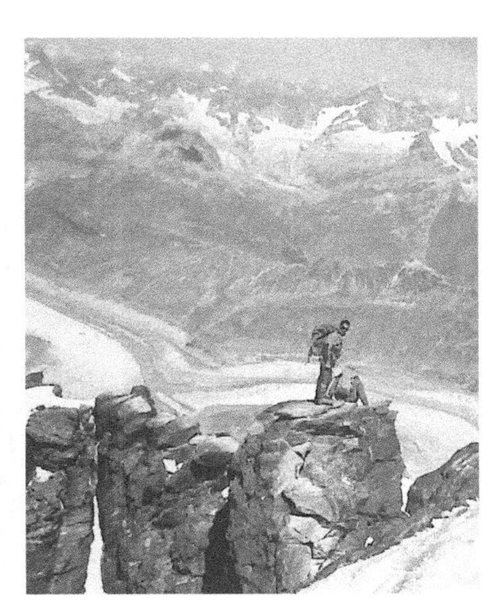

I have an innate need for perspective and heightened experiences. It is a hunger that can only be fed by exploring these places for myself. The lessons I've brought back from these experiences have changed my life, and now, have found their way onto these pages.

## Perspective from Chimborazo, Ecuador

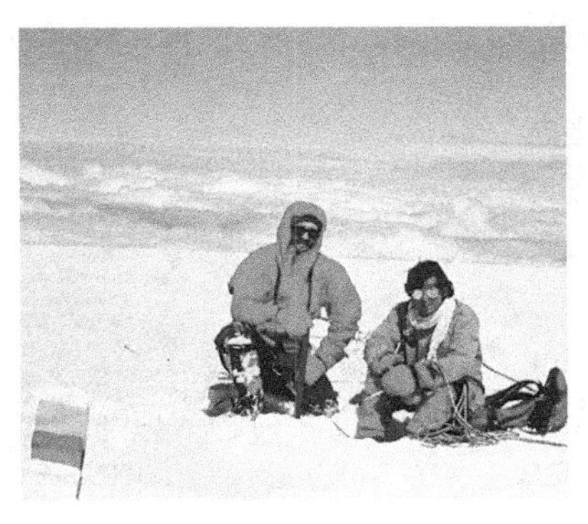

"A mind, once expanded by new ideas, never returns to its original dimensions." Oliver Wendell Holmes

I've been lucky to be able to stand atop tall peaks all around the world. I learn something important with every hike, every climb.

Until the beginning of the 19th century, Chimborazo was thought to be the highest mountain on Earth. While that was proven untrue, the equatorial bulge on our planet gives this summit a geologic and geographic distinction: it is the farthest point away from the center of the Earth. A most unusual place to gain a dose of both heightened perspective and deep humility.

## Atop Mont Blanc, Chamonix, France

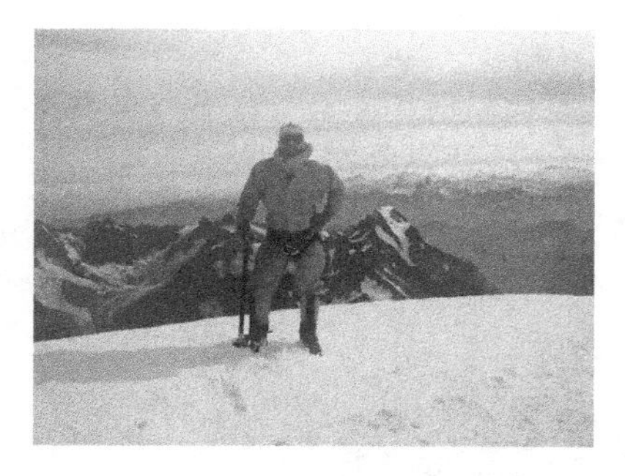

This is one of my favorite summits in the world, with a commanding view across all of Europe. I've been there five times. Each time, I'm aware of the Matterhorn, tiny and far off on the horizon. Mont Blanc is where modern mountaineering began in the 1770s. Hiking and climbing the surrounding hills were my first stops as I broadened my international travels.

## Climbing the Matterhorn

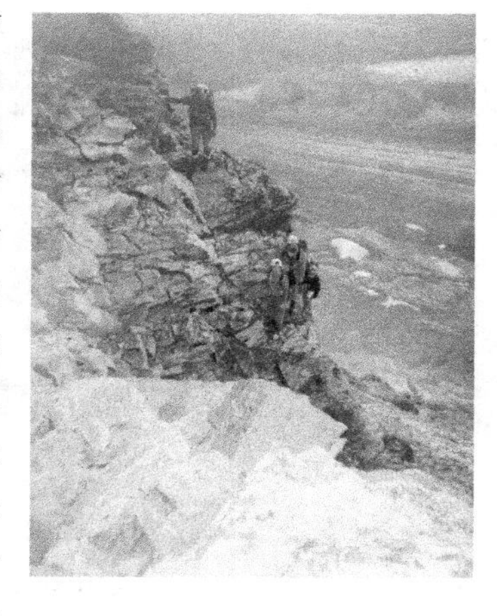

The Matterhorn has been my fascination since childhood—an inspiration and a motivator. It has been the driving symbol of my business career and the muse for my transformation from the corporate to the entrepreneurial world. It's also been the rationale for this book.

Climbing it is the equivalent of a 5,000-foot rock ladder. But like solving any difficult or scary problem, you acquire the skills to do this layer by layer—starting small, gaining experience, taking a few risks, and working your way forward. Eventually, you have both the mental and physical abilities to succeed. These valuable life lessons are scattered across many chapters of the book.

## Halfway Up the Matterhorn

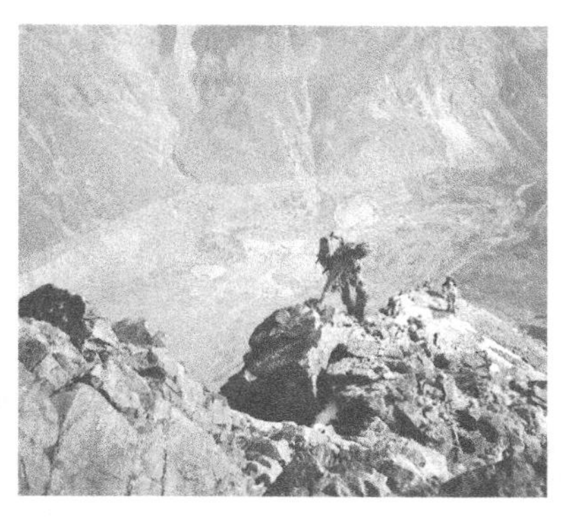

Here you are exposed on a knife-edged ridge with thousands of feet down on either side of you. You become increasingly aware that you have to climb back down this ladder. It can be daunting and dizzying if you think too much about the drop-off.

It's an extreme example, but an excellent demonstration that many of the challenges we face are mental challenges. You begin with smaller tests, and you teach yourself to focus your thoughts on the present moment, blocking out all distractions. You learn self-reliance, and you learn persistence. And before you know it, you can overcome obstacles you once thought impossible.

## Looking Down from the Top

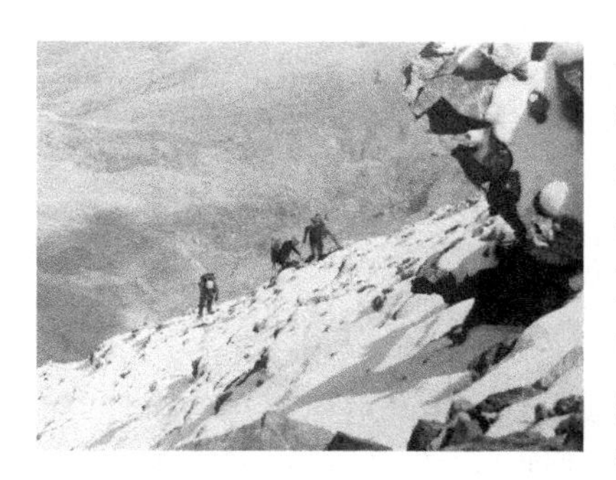

As I sat on the pointy summit of the Matterhorn collecting my thoughts and preparing for the equally difficult descent, I was already thinking about the future. Achieving a lofty goal, especially one that takes a great deal of time and effort to achieve, leads one to the obvious question: "What next?" I've always appreciated the significance of this simple Zen parable, "When you get to the top of the mountain, keep climbing." So, that's the answer. You find another goal, another mountain. As a result, I decided my motto is, "Always seeking another summit." I intend never to stop heading uphill. See Chapter 19.

## Stretch Your Comfort Zone

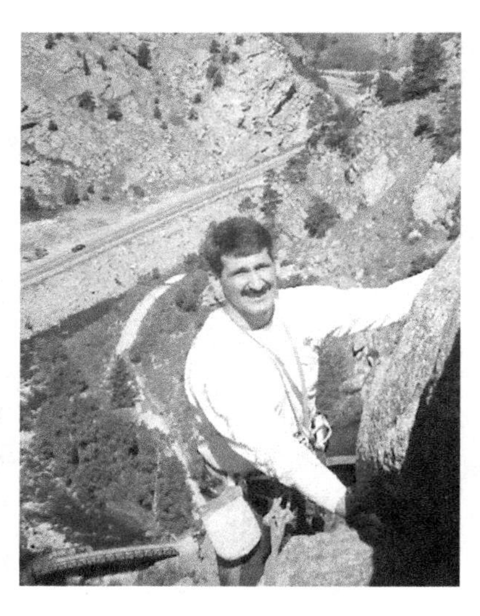

If you want to grow, you have to take a risk. You have to stretch. You have to fall and fail along the way.

I get antsy unless I'm trying to stretch my comfort zone. I feel like things are too easy. I feel like I'm not making progress.

But sometimes you can push too far. On this crag in Boulder, Colorado, I discovered my limitations. When you are faced with these choices and challenges in life, you must make a decision. Is pushing forward worthwhile, or do your skills and interests lie elsewhere? See Chapter 11.

## Find Your Own Peak

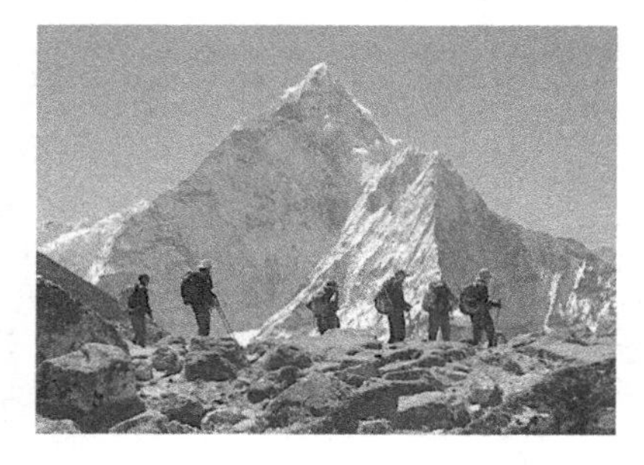

You do not have to become a mountaineer to learn these lessons. You do not have risk life and limb to experience profound changes in your fitness level, your brain health, your healthspan, and your spirit. So many great adventures are accessible to you if you choose to take the first steps—walk, start an exercise program, go for a hike, and go higher if you like. Many people I've met along the trails, in the hills, and on the great mountains of the world have done just that. You will never know where walking uphill will take you until you get outside and try it for yourself.

---

*"Whatever you can dream you can do, begin it. Boldness has genius and power and magic in it."*

**– Johann Wolfgang von Goethe**

---

You'll find more stories, pictures, and inspiration at **GetOutside.online.**

SECTION 3

# The Fitness You Can't Get in a Gym

# 10

# THERE'S SOMETHING ABOUT MOUNTAINS

*So if you cannot understand that there is something in man which responds to the challenge of this mountain and goes out to meet it, that the struggle is the struggle of life itself, then you won't see why we go. What we get from this adventure is just sheer joy. And joy is, after all, the end of life. We do not live to eat and make money. We eat and make money to be able to enjoy life. That is what life means and what life is for.*

— GEORGE LEIGH MALLORY,
EARLY MOUNT EVEREST PIONEER

There's something about mountains that is built into the human psyche: they symbolize big goals, lofty dreams and aspirations, difficult challenges, and strength. As Mallory said, they are the perfect metaphor for the struggle of life itself. We see this everywhere we look. Quite frequently, mountains are used as logos. Think Prudential insurance, Coors beer, Toblerone chocolate, Paramount movie studio, and countless small businesses around the world—all hoping to connote substance, solidity, presence, power.

But beyond the symbolism, there are many lessons to be learned in the mountains, available to anyone willing to go. Merely getting up close to big mountains, at the base, or from the valley below, you can feel their power and inspiration. It may even serve as a temptation to get closer and higher.

In this chapter, I hope to help you find your own inspiration—what you aspire to accomplish. You'll see from my story that I started small and built up to the high peaks. You can do it, too.

What is the first thing you think when you see a tall mountain? Do you think it majestic and pretty? Or do you think it cold, inhospitable, or even sinister? Does it provoke inspiration and awe, or fear and avoidance?

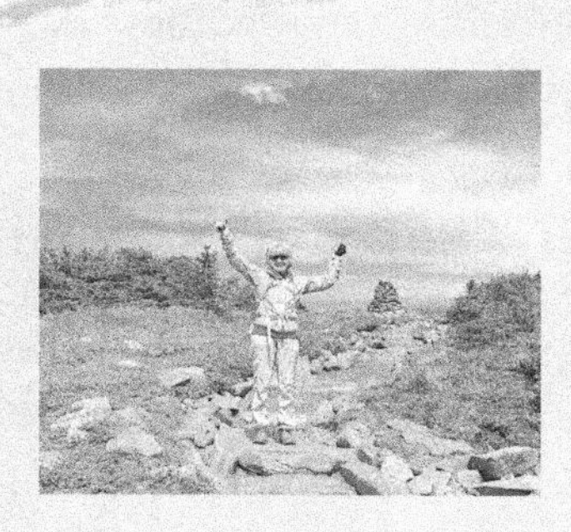

"It was amazing—the sensory overload of wind, vista, space, exhilaration. What have I been missing my whole life? I'm going to do more of this!"

- Susan Williams,
from Connecticut, discovered hiking at age 45. Now 73 and as fit as ever.

Until the early part of the 1800s, mountains were thought to be forbidden, evil, haunted places. Knowledge of how mountains were formed was decidedly inaccurate, and most of the world's biggest mountains had barely been seen, much less explored or climbed. The Himalayas, the Andes, the Rockies, and Africa's Kilimanjaro were unknown, mysterious places to most of the people on the planet. Can you imagine there was once a world with no photography and no Instagram? What they did think about mountains was mostly negative, if they thought about them at all: hostile, treacherous, unnatural—the province of beasts, spirits, and nightmares.

But human nature being what it is, eventually, curiosity won out. The spirit of exploration that was sweeping across Europe and North America in the 1800s led braver souls to look up and venture into these unknown places. Much of this activity centered on the Alps in France and Switzerland, and the years 1850–1890 became known as The Golden Age of Mountaineering. Climbers from all over the world, mostly European, went to the Alps, and over those few decades, every summit above 12,000 feet was reached. Thus, the sport of mountaineering was born.

## How I Fell in Love with the Mountains

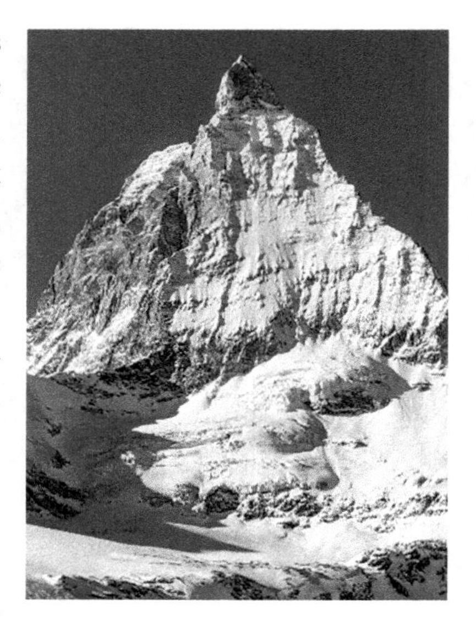

This is the Matterhorn. It was the ultimate prize during the golden age of mountaineering, and I have been in love with it since I saw its picture at age six, and again in the Disney movie *Third Man on the Mountain*. (This movie is why there is a Matterhorn at Disneyland in Anaheim.)

My first thought when seeing a picture of it was simple. Pretty much, "Wow!!??" But right after that, it was, "I wonder what the world looks like from up there?" I was powerfully drawn to it. From that point on, I began a lifelong pursuit of the remote high places of the world, and a never-ending need to know,

"What does the world look like from up there?" (I do this with tall buildings too.)

I suppose for me, it is an innate search for perspective and heightened experiences. It is a hunger that could only be fed by exploring these places for myself. Little did I realize at the time, but it has been the driving symbol of my business career, my inevitable transition from the corporate to the entrepreneurial world, and the rationale for this book.

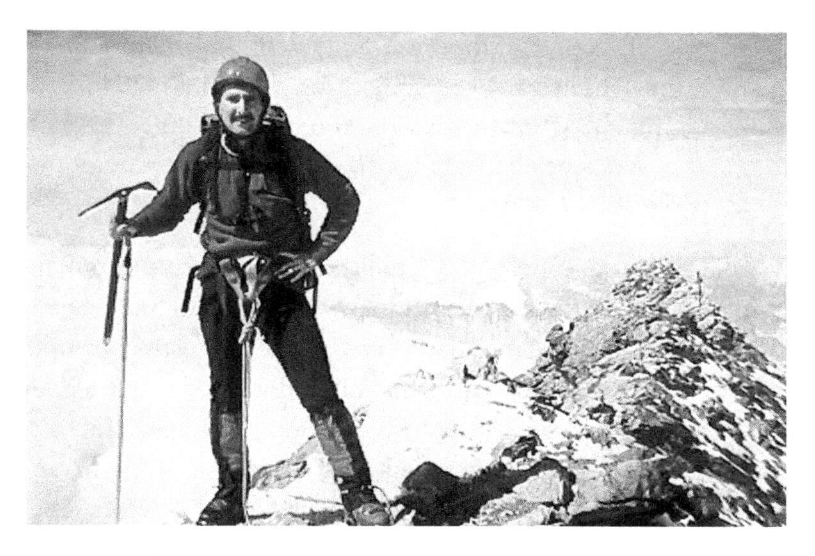

So, this is me on top of the Matterhorn, about 25 years later. Goal achieved. It was worth the wait, and it was everything I had hoped it would be. Life-changing. Energizing. There's a saying that "your mind, once expanded, can never go back to its old dimensions," and this was certainly the case for me. It's also said that at the tops of some mountains, particularly those with very narrow, pointed peaks, the universe is able to focus its energy on those lofty spots, allowing you to absorb that energy when you stand there. It does feel that way sometimes. It was so profound I couldn't even put into words what I was feeling.

The only thing that ever came close to describing it was Rob Schultheis in *Bone Games:*

> Imagine that someone, a terrible wizard, gave you a potion that made everything perfect for a few hours; you knew everything, you could do anything, all your dreams come true. Then the potion wore off and you found yourself back in your old, tired out body with your old, ignorant mind. The wizard has gone away, no one knows where, taking his potions with him. You had tasted heaven, now you were stuck back on earth, with no sign of redemption *(Schultheis 1986).*

I did have that experience. And it was so addictive it took me back to the top of the Matterhorn four more times to find it again.

I've discovered the mountains are wonderful testing grounds and teachers. They teach you who you really are if you are open to their many lessons. And they are nature's fitness club and mindfulness program, a never-ending source of strength and inspiration for body and mind—a playground for adults. They have shaped my career and my life in innumerable ways.

## I Really Do Love Mountains

As I mentioned, despite being born in very flat and unmistakably non-remote Brooklyn and living my first decade in equally flat and sea-level Queens, New York, and Bergenfield, New Jersey, I've been powerfully drawn to mountains from a very early age. I suppose it was the contrast that appealed to me: flat and man-made versus tall, pointy, and totally random and wild.

When I went to the library, it was to read about Sir Edmund Hillary, Jim Whittaker, and Tom Hornbein climbing Mount Everest, or Thor Heyerdahl exploring Easter Island, or Apollo astronauts on the Moon. I was riveted by Robert F. Kennedy's climb of Canada's Mount Kennedy in 1969—the very first ascent, to honor his assassinated brother. It revealed that climbing mountains is more than an athletic feat and that there is great symbolism and meaning in achieving a summit.

Little did I know at age 12 that this curiosity would be a powerful motivator spurring me on, not just to the Matterhorn but to explore all four corners of the earth, from Antarctica to Everest. It transformed me from a city kid and book smart junior executive to a seasoned global executive and adventurer who prefers a tent or a mountain hut to a suite at The Mandarin Oriental Hotel in Hong Kong (not surprisingly, every time I've been to Hong Kong, I've been compelled to go up to the top of Victoria Peak for that amazing 360° view).

We moved from metro New York to "hill country" Connecticut in 1968. Upon arriving, my dad immediately started a Boy Scout troop for my brother and me, and the whole neighborhood got behind it. This is when the outdoors really began to call to me. We lived at the top of a small, wooded mountain with a view for miles and miles. We camped in the backyard, hiked in the nearby woods, built a kid-powered dogsled to compete in the Klondike

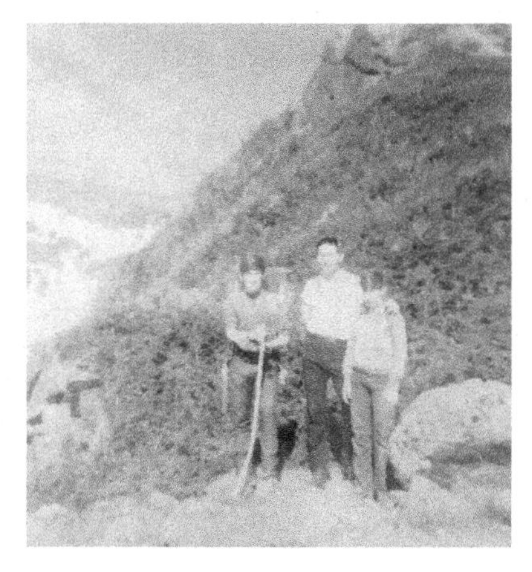

*On Lion Head Trail*

Derby at Camp Mattatuck, and spent summer vacations in New Hampshire campgrounds.

And that's where I got my first look at Mount Washington, the highest peak in the Northeast. Though it is a mere 6,288 feet above sea level and diminutive by global standards, it is still a legitimate mountain, with Antarctic-like weather in winter, massive glacial bowls and ridges, remote wilderness trails, and a summit well above tree-line.

In 1971, I finally got to go there. My dad took my brother Michael and me to stay at the Joe Dodge Lodge in Pinkham Notch. The next day, we hiked up to the Hermit Lake Shelters and into the massive glacial cirque of Tuckerman Ravine. The following day, we climbed to the summit up the Lion Head Trail. I loved every second of it. I didn't want to leave. The memory of it—snow in June, the vast expanse above treeline, the rugged trails with very few people—all almost as clear in my mind as the reality of it was nearly fifty years ago.

A few years later, I braved it again, this time

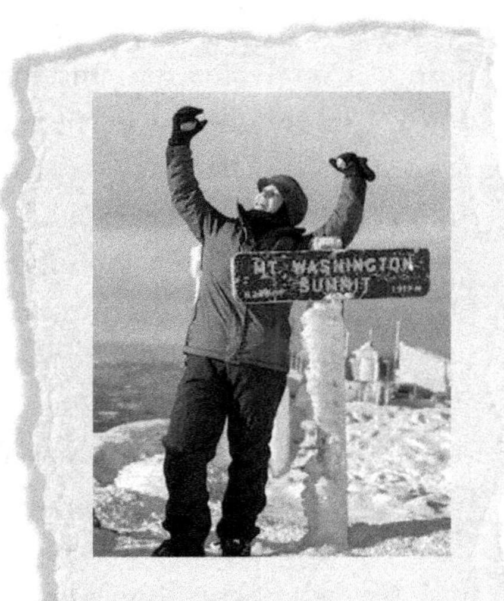


This is Sandy Sherman from Vermont, who began hiking just ten years ago. She's a small business owner, mom, and cancer survivor, who has now, at age 54, hiked the 67 tallest peaks in New England and inspired many people along the way. "Magic moments happen all the time in the mountains. I feel honored to witness some of the sights I've seen through the years. You will gain perspective, expand your thinking, and experience awe."

with some high school friends in late winter, and we had an epic adventure where we froze our butts off in a snow cave shelter. We skied Tuckerman's Ravine and the summit snowfields, and we almost fell through the ice into a raging torrent of meltwater. Again, I couldn't get enough of it. I was hooked—deeply—and not just on the physical nature of the experience. I could sense there was indeed a serious mental and spiritual aspect to this that I couldn't verbalize at the time. It was an overwhelming sensory infusion that was powerful, magical, and addictive. I needed more.

## So, I Became a Mountaineer

In my 20s and 30s, I set my heights higher. Squeezed into a demanding business career, I became a mountaineer. I had designs on finishing the Seven Summits (climbing the tallest peak on each continent) and getting to the top of Everest when relatively few people had been there—long before it was a crowded, guided undertaking.

So, I began to train and add skills, layer by layer, with the challenges increasing incrementally, in difficulty and in duration. First, there was Mount Rainier, which at 14,410 feet is one of the best training grounds for aspiring high-altitude mountaineers. While training for it, I did a solo winter climb of Mount Washington and met another solo climber, far more experienced than I on the summit, where it was below zero and quite windy. Taking shelter together in an alcove near the summit weather station, he offered advice: "You must go to Rainier. That's where all the Everest climbers are." That's all I needed to hear. I climbed it five times in just a few years and learned technique and experience from some of the best high-altitude climbers in the world.

Then I moved on to the Alps, rock climbing in Boulder, Colorado, and the Rockies, all the Mexican volcanoes, Antarctica, Ecuador, Africa, Alaska, and more. A LOT of uphill steps, a lot of outdoor mileage, a lot of training for it all, and recently, a lot of learning about the significance of meeting that 75-year-old trail runner on Mount Washington.

Since then, hiking and climbing have taken me to all seven continents. But you do not have to take it to this level. I've met plenty of people who know what I know and are far more skilled than I, who got the same benefits I did while never leaving their home states of New Hampshire, or Colorado, or Oregon.

As it turned out, the Matterhorn is my inspiration and motivation. It's my peak, and it happens to be an actual mountain. But yours doesn't have to be. A peak is any goal you set your sights on. You must find your own peak.

# 11

# STRETCH YOUR COMFORT ZONE

*The mountains reserve their choice gifts for those who stand upon their summits.*

— SIR FRANCES YOUNGHUSBAND

If you want to grow, to learn, to improve, you have to take a risk. You have to stretch. You have to fall and fail along the way.

I'm sure you've heard the oft-repeated saying that regularly makes the rounds of social media: "Life begins at the end of your comfort zone." That popular quote was preceded by the quote that begins the chapter, attributed to Sir Francis Younghusband, who was a British explorer of the late 1800s. Long before Younghusband, ancient philosophers said essentially the same thing. It is part of the human condition, so you might as well accept it. There is no escaping the fact that to improve at anything, to receive those choice gifts, you have to constantly be pushing against the limits of your abilities.

Do you recall when you made the leap from a tricycle to a two-wheeler? Then to a ten-speed bike? Each new level seemed hard, paralyzing. You worried about losing your balance and falling, so you used training wheels to help, and then you broke through and got comfortable with the next level. That's what we're talking about. First, you crawl, then you walk, then you jog, then you run, and then you sprint. For some reason, those very simple childhood lessons don't seem to stick with us into adulthood, and we often have to relearn them. If we don't, we risk crawling into a comfortable little comfort zone.

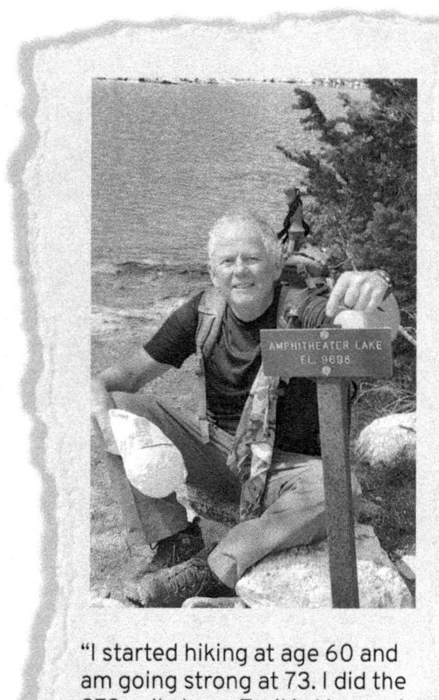


"I started hiking at age 60 and am going strong at 73. I did the 273-mile Long Trail in Vermont, end to end. Hiked and rafted the Grand Canyon, hiked in the Tetons and High Sierras, and will be hiking around Moab this coming April. Hiking has changed my life for the better in many ways."

– Keld Alstrup, Vermont

Fitness, exercising, getting outside, and hiking are extremely well-suited ways to relearn that lesson as adults. You have opportunities to set goals, take small steps towards your goals, and have fun along the way. But, more importantly, you have the opportunity to make it stick, to turn a healthy lifestyle into a habit that increases your chances of living a long, happy, healthy life.

## Comfort Zones Are a Trap

A comfort zone is a place where you feel safe, familiar, and cozy. A place where, sing it, "Everybody knows your name." There are no obstacles in your comfort zone. No risk. You can pull the covers up over your eyes and block out the world. You can live vicariously through others or through YouTube. Safe is good, right? Well, no, not necessarily.

When you are at ease, unstressed, and protected, it's very alluring. It can be restful and comfortable on a comfy couch, in your office, or in your safe space. It can be seductive and addictive. But living perpetually in your comfort zone makes you complacent and overly content that all is well. I don't think we are on this planet to sit passively and do little or nothing. Which means you've got to get up, get out into the world, and take action. Use what you're given, find your potential, and engage. That means you've got to take a risk.

A place without stress is also a place of no growth. Your first Spanish lesson was scary, right? Your first piano lesson was daunting too. Math is scary, right? Your first time at the gym was probably confusing and intimidating. Your first hike in the woods and hills might be that way too. That's just the way it works.

Muscles respond to stress by growing larger. Bones respond to stress by building new cells that make them stronger. And if they do break, the healed spot is stronger than the surrounding bone. Your body builds endurance and strength through stress. Your heart gets stronger when you make it work increasingly harder, stressing it a bit. Your brain responds to learning and stimulation (i.e., stress) by growing new neural pathways. You build the neural pathways that make up an effortless tennis serve by sucking at it for a long time. You build the skills to recognize and hit a curveball by watching and swinging at 10,000 curveballs and missing 8,500 of them. You build the skills to climb a tall mountain by walking first, then hiking, then climbing small mountains, then higher mountains. Each level upward is a new expansion of your comfort zone.

## Comfort Zones: Big versus Small

Your psyche also benefits from the stress of exiting your comfort zone and trying something new.

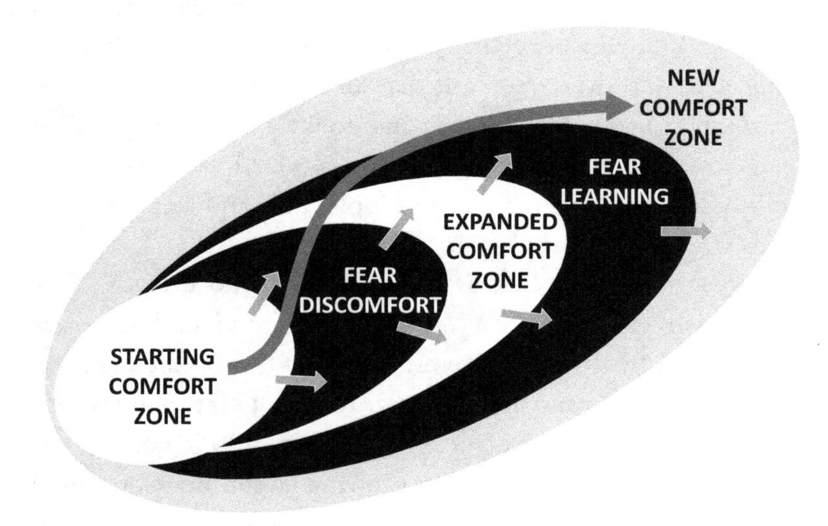


Like a lot of people who have gravitated toward hiking, trekking, and climbing, I get antsy unless I'm trying to stretch my comfort zone. I feel like things are too easy. I feel like I'm not making progress. If I'm too comfortable, I can't always describe what progress I should or want to be making, but I'm left feeling like I am underperforming. I won't deny it. From time to time, it is great to feel safe and protected. But sooner or later, I've got to put myself out there, whether it is the physical challenge of hiking and climbing or my work as an entrepreneur. I am compelled not to play it safe, but to test myself and try to do something worthwhile and difficult.

Not surprisingly, I had an instinctive feeling that I should be passing these values on to my son Michael. Of course, I chose the outdoors as our classroom. At an early age, he became a very willing accomplice to some of my adventures. I was pretty sure he was capable because youth soccer and basketball had him running year-round, and I knew he was aerobically fit.

So, without any preliminary minor hikes, at age seven, he climbed Mount Washington with me. I don't think he broke a sweat. Then we did a much harder Presidential Traverse across the entire range and then Huntington Ravine on Mount Washington, the most difficult trail in the White Mountains—no sweat, no fear, no complaints. Kids are like that. The lessons of crawl, walk, jog, run, sprint and tricycle, bicycle, ten-speed are still fresh in their minds. Better yet, they don't know there's such a thing as a comfort zone if you don't tell them.

I took him rock climbing in Boulder, Colorado, and he scampered up the Flatirons without any difficulty. Wow, kids are incredible, natural, and fearless climbers! This went on for a few years until I felt certain he was a very capable and confident hiker. Next up, I wanted to expand his world in a big way with a much bigger risk, so we decided to climb Mount Kilimanjaro in Africa when he was 13.

Kilimanjaro lies on the border between Kenya and Tanzania. At 19,340 feet, it is the highest point in Africa and one of the fabled Seven Summits. It is the remnant of an ancient and much larger super-volcano that collapsed into itself and is now a gargantuan pile of rubble with fifteen separate glaciers on top, the legendary "Snows of Kilimanjaro."

As climbs go, Kilimanjaro is mostly a long, tedious, very scenic, uphill hike. It starts out in a tropical jungle and passes through every variation of climate zone on earth up to the arctic/polar summit. It's five long days of uphill on the Machame Route, far from the tourists rushing up the other side of the mountain. It's quite a grind.

The big challenge when climbing Kilimanjaro is acclimatizing to the high altitude. The higher up you go, the less oxygen there is in the air. Your body needs time to adapt to the lower oxygen levels. At nearly 20,000 feet, there is less than 60 percent of the oxygen available to you that you would have at sea level. This stresses your body and forces it to create new red blood cells. Those new cells supply your muscles and brain with adequate oxygen to offset the altitude. This process is a perfect physiological example of how stressing your body (i.e., getting out of your comfort zone) encourages adaptation to a new, higher level. Frankly, I think my son had less trouble with the altitude than I did.

When we crested the volcano's crater rim at the summit, it was quite a moment. We weren't home and safe yet, but I was immensely relieved. I had assured my skeptical, but in the end, trusting wife that he would be perfectly capable of doing this, and we could get him up and down the mountain safely. It's kind of risky taking a 13-year-old to the top of Kilimanjaro, but in the end, it turned out to have been a life-changing, mega-experience that reinforced for both of us the concept of aiming high and taking calculated risks out of your comfort zone.

This shot has become the money shot from our trip. Shortly before turning in at Barafu high camp (at about 16,000 feet) on the eve of our summit climb, my son wandered over to the edge of a drop-off to survey the sunset. How often does a 13-year-old kid get to look out across central Africa from above the clouds? Mind properly expanded, never to go back to its old dimensions, I thought.

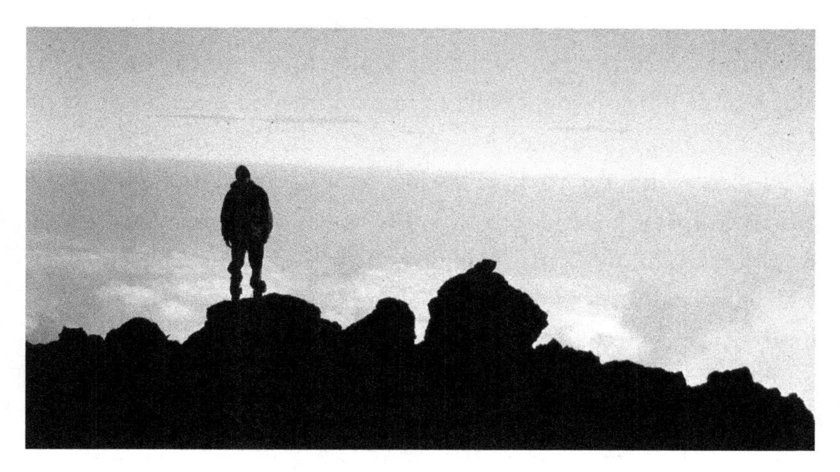

It must have worked because more than 20 years later, he is an entrepreneur and investment banker, and along with his wife, also an entrepreneur and hiker. They recently completed the legendary Haute Route, an extremely difficult 75-mile mountain trek from Mont Blanc, Chamonix, France, to the Matterhorn in Zermatt, Switzerland. Not surprisingly, they have chosen to live amongst the mountains of the Pacific Northwest.

## Pushing Past Your Comfort Zone

As you get more experience with the idea of getting out of your comfort zone, you get more comfortable with what you can and cannot do. You learn to balance not just the risks of a situation, but what you're willing to risk. There's no rule that says you have to keep pushing your hardest on everything. You can decide when you want to move forward and when you want to change direction.

One of the first times I discovered the power of this choice was as I began to explore the tallest mountains of the world. I realized it might be important to be both an accomplished mountaineer and a technical rock climber. Since the Matterhorn was my obsession, and it's a 5,000-foot rock ridge, I knew I needed a certain level of rock-climbing confidence to get safely to the summit.

I began taking rock climbing lessons from the guides in North Conway, New Hampshire, in the Pacific Northwest, and in Boulder, Colorado. I made progress, but I quickly realized there were physical limitations to my abilities. The best rock climbers tend to be built like gymnasts, extremely lean with amazing upper-body strength. I'm built the other way—more of a bull or yak than a chimpanzee or gazelle. I'm very good going long distances while carrying a heavy pack or pulling a sled of supplies up a mountain and less suited to going up a vertical rock wall. But I was going to try to get better.

Cut to Boulder Canyon in Colorado. I was climbing with Duncan Ferguson, a rock-climbing guide. It was probably the third time I had climbed with him. We had previously done easier climbs and routes, but I was gaining confidence, so we decided I was ready to push it a little.

I was roped to him, and he was leading the way. Several hundred feet up the near-vertical cliff, we came upon a little bulge-overhang. If it had been at ground level, I would not have given it a second thought. But here, several hundred feet up, I could not get my body to reach out and back to grab an easy handhold. Even though I was roped up and fairly protected by his secure belay, I could not do it. I froze.

Just as I was thinking this through, another climber came into view directly below us. He was free soloing the same route we were on—unroped and moving three times as fast as me. He was practically running up a cliff where one misstep would result in a fatal fall. When he reached us, he paused for a second, said hello (Duncan knew him), and climbed past the exact spot where I was frozen. Here was a person not only of greater ability but also in a completely different mental space. This amount of vertical was not as steep or as high to him. The risk I could not wrap my head around, the reach back and around that I could not force myself to do, well, he didn't hesitate for a second. He made that move as if he had done it 1,000 times before because he probably had. Then off he went, up and out of sight.

Well, that was it for me. On that day, I knew I had reached a point where it was not the physical part of climbing that was holding me back. It was what was going on in my head. I decided it was time to back off and get my head right. We rappelled back to the ground and called it a day. I had work to do if I wanted to get to the next level.

I thought about that moment a great deal. With additional practice and training, I knew I could probably overcome that obstacle and make the reach that had paralyzed me before. But I was also aware I was never going to be a high-level rock climber because of my physique. As far as rock climbing goes, I was going to peak in a very mediocre place. I had a choice to make. Fortunately, I felt pretty good about the level I had reached. While it was not good enough for the elite big wall like the rock climbs you find in places like Yosemite, it was good enough for the Matterhorn and many other exciting, tall mountains in the world. And guess what? I was (and still am) okay with that. I'll push my comfort zone elsewhere.

That's the beauty of comfort zones. You discover and explore limits. Then, you decide what's important and where you want to focus your energy. The process typically involves making small choices and decisions along the way. Each of these actions collectively gives you the confidence to try bigger things. Although this seems a basic concept, it is one best learned by living and internalizing experiences. That confidence breeds additional confidence until a certain self-efficacy becomes the norm. You are confident that whatever comes up, whatever obstacles, distractions, setbacks hit you, you will thrive and succeed. It's infectious.

As you get more experience with this concept of getting out of your comfort zone, you get more comfortable with what you can and cannot do, but also what you're willing to risk. There's no rule that says you have to keep pushing forward on everything. You decide what is worth it and what can wait for another day.

My recommendation? Make a plan to get out of your comfort zone at least once a month (or once a week if you're up for it). Stretch yourself a little bit, and you'll be surprised how much you grow.

---

*"Always in the big woods when you leave familiar ground and step off alone into a new place there will be, along with feelings of curiosity and excitement, a little nagging of dread. It is fear of the Unknown, and it is your first bond with the wilderness you are going into. What you are doing is exploring. You are undertaking the first experience, not of the place, but of yourself in that place."*

**- Wendell Berry**

---

# 12

# FIND YOUR OWN PEAK

*If you have built castles in the air, your work need not be lost; that is where they should be. Now put the foundations under them."*

— HENRY DAVID THOREAU

My castles—my goals—have always been in the air. One became a lifelong obsession. At an age when I had absolutely no clue about how to attain it or what skills I would need or even how to begin, my peak was the Matterhorn.

It took me 25 years to achieve it. And it has led to other goals, other peaks, and instilled me with a sense that when faced with daunting challenges and obstacles, they can almost always be overcome if you are willing to begin by taking the first small steps. The important thing is to begin, and from there, things unfold in ways you cannot possibly imagine if you don't take that first step.

I want to impress on you that not every challenge has to be a tall mountain. People face their own stubborn, discouraging, daunting, seemingly mountainous obstacles everywhere in life.

Your mountain doesn't have to be my mountain. It doesn't have to be a big one. It doesn't even have to be a mountain. And you don't have to go to the top. I get it that mountains, uphill, remote places, etc. can be daunting and scary. So, it can be a dream, a wish, a plan. Mountains are merely a metaphor for a goal.

## Finding My Peak

My first climb of the Matterhorn, my lifelong obsession, is a story of setbacks, overcoming fear, mental challenges, turning points, and great joy.

It's 2:00 a.m. I'm standing with 20 other climbers at the base of the first section of a 5,000-foot-tall vertical ridge. The first 25 feet are almost straight up, but fairly easy because there are big handholds and footholds, like a ladder. We'd all just been woken up in the Hornli Hut at the base of the ridge, crammed down a quick breakfast, and raced up the trail to this spot. We were roped together in groups of twos and threes, headlamps ablaze in the dark, breath visible in the frigid air, waiting for the first few climbers to get up and through this little bottleneck right at the start.

My turn. I move up to the first step, onto the mountain I had waited my whole life to climb. I placed my right foot 18 inches up onto this easy step, reached up for the handhold, and my boot skidded off on the rime-iced foothold. I slipped on the first step of a 5,000-foot ladder of rock. I looked down at my foot, and in three seconds, waves of panic, self-doubt, and fear of failure popped into my head: "I can't do this. What will the rest of the mountain be like! I'm not supposed to be here. Maybe I should go back to the hut and forget about this nonsense."

On the fourth second, my rope mate, already 25 feet up, gives the rope a tug. I take a deep breath, look at the Swiss guide waiting his turn right behind me, nodding "Go." I squelched the panic and climbed up the pitch without incident.

Cut to four hours later. I am about halfway up the 5,000-foot ridge at a very steep section called Moseley Platte, named for an American climber who fell to his death from the spot in 1879. I have about 20 feet to go before it levels off and gets easier and safer, and that same pesky right boot could not get a good foothold and was flailing around for grip. I'm hanging on, knowing full well the significance of the Moseley Platte. I can't find the next step and again think, "I can't do it. I'm not supposed to be here!"

Suddenly, I feel a force firmly place my boot about a foot to the right. I look down through my legs at my feet, and I see that same Swiss guide. He had grabbed my heel and guided my foot, which was pretty much in his face, to the proper position. "Danke," I said. "Bitte," he replied. And I continued upward. Again, I was made aware of the significance of a single step, and the idea that from time to time, a nudge in the right direction is all you need to overcome the doubt, to keep going.

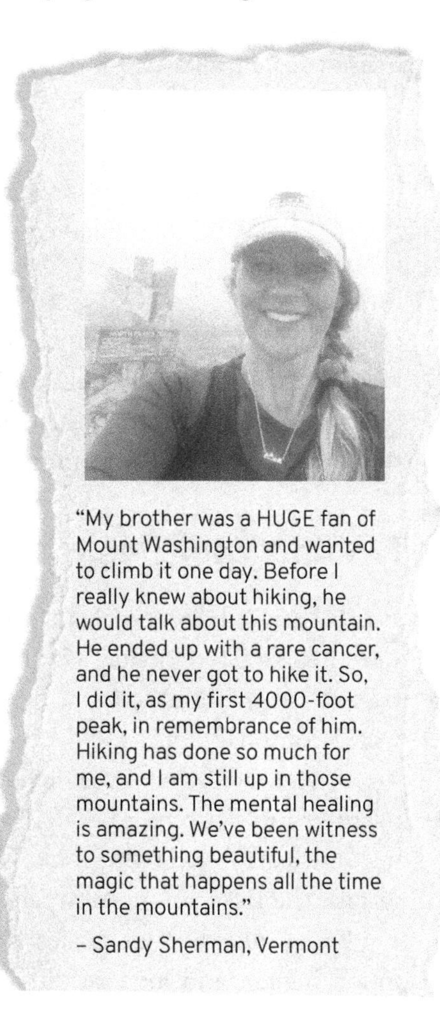

"My brother was a HUGE fan of Mount Washington and wanted to climb it one day. Before I really knew about hiking, he would talk about this mountain. He ended up with a rare cancer, and he never got to hike it. So, I did it, as my first 4000-foot peak, in remembrance of him. Hiking has done so much for me, and I am still up in those mountains. The mental healing is amazing. We've been witness to something beautiful, the magic that happens all the time in the mountains."

– Sandy Sherman, Vermont

Now cut to another four hours later. I am sitting, exhausted, on the summit of the Matterhorn, a bit in disbelief that I am actually there. I look up, and cresting the final steps is that same Swiss guide, pulling his client up behind him. They'd pretty much followed me the whole way up. As he came to where I was sitting, this seasoned, grizzled climbing guide who had probably dragged hundreds of climbers to that spot over the years, tapped my helmet as he walked by and said, "Nice job."

The moment is still fresh in my head thirty years later. And not only does it speak to the importance of taking the first steps, but it also speaks to how a simple human moment and a few words of encouragement can be deeply felt, motivating, and even unforgettable. Fitness trainers and coaches: please never forget this.

I think of this climb, and those small moments often, when faced with moments of doubt against other challenges, and I recall that if I could get through that slip on the first step and the rest of that day, I could deal with most anything that came my way.

## Finding Your Peak

When I am outside, especially in the mountains, I breathe better; I see better; I feel better. My mind is clearer, and I think better. I don't ruminate about the never-ending problems in the real world. I am happier.

If you don't get outside enough, your thinking becomes narrow, and your mind leans towards scarcity. As a result, you become fearful and risk-averse. You may not be proactive enough or take the risks you need to take.

Being outside a lot makes you feel part of something much, much bigger, and as a result, you'll see the world through an abundance mindset, believing there are unlimited possibilities. Your thinking expands because you see that the world is so much larger than you.

For me, it can be distilled down to joy. That's what getting outside is for me, and I suspect you can get that feeling too because it is available right outside your door. You don't have to climb the Matterhorn to get a big helping of joy.

I believe the mountains made me; they made me an entrepreneur by making me willing to accept a much higher degree of risk and personal responsibility than I had when I was a big corporate animal. They made me stronger, more confident, more worldly, more seasoned, and certainly wiser. They can do that for you too. Maybe your goal isn't entrepreneurial, but that's not the point. The challenges and mind expansion that come with getting outside will translate to confidence and increased clarity in all aspects of life.

So, my advice is to get out there and find your own peak. Things really do look different from "up there."

---

*"And then it hits you. You are not in the mountains; the mountains are in you."*

**– John Muir**

---

# 13

# HIKING PUTS THE BRAIN FIRST

*I often tell my patients that the point of exercise is to build and condition the brain.*

— DR. JOHN RATEY

The brain uses about 20 to 30 percent of the nutrients you ingest and the oxygen you breathe, even though it weighs only four pounds. It is the neediest of all organs, and since it controls every movement you make, every sensation you feel, every thought you have, and every other organ in your body, brain health must come first.

Brain health and body health are not mutually exclusive. Brain health is body health. If you make brain health the priority for the way you approach fitness, the body follows.

And here is an important and related concept to consider: stop thinking about lifespan as a single, narrow goal. Your health span is what is really important—the number of years you live in good health, where you are mobile, self-sufficient, and clear of mind. A major part of why we should seek improved fitness is to make sure your brain lasts as long as your body. I can think of few things worse than slipping into dementia or Alzheimer's while the rest of your body is still working fine.

So, if you are above age 45, now is the time to adopt a brain-first attitude and a brain-healthy lifestyle. The consequence of ignoring this is the furthering of one of the single most significant health problems we will face in the next 100 years: exponential increases in dementia, Parkinson's, and Alzheimer's, due to an aging, inactive population. It appears that much of this can be prevented with lifestyle changes that involve certain kinds of brain-healthy exercise.

I was taught to believe, like everyone else, that we were all born with a finite number of brain cells, and those cells were the only brain cells we were ever going to have. And that as you aged, smoked cigarettes, drank alcohol, were put under great stress, or slept poorly (or became a boxer or football player and were repeatedly pounded on the head), you were killing brain cells that could never be restored. Excess drinking even became known in the vernacular as "killing brain cells." Old boxers were referred to as punch drunk.

As it turns out, all those things are still terribly bad for your brain, but that is only half the story.

In the mid-90s, it was discovered that brain cells—neurons—could be regenerated in adult brains. While studying mice on a treadmill, scientists discovered neuron growth in the hippocampus, the part of the brain responsible for memory. Additional studies have since shown this works on humans as well, and at present, there is clear evidence that certain kinds of exercise and cognitive challenges can build new brain cells in adult brains of any age. The process of creating new neurons, new brain cells, is called neurogenesis.

And contrary to what you may suspect, it is not that hard to make neurogenesis happen. Recent learning suggests that neurogenesis is a normal, built-in system to protect and repair the brain, much like stem cells work with bone marrow and skin (Society for Neuroscience 2020). Under the right conditions, neurogenesis is a natural process available to anyone.

What are those right conditions? Primarily, the physical activity we call, drumroll please, EXERCISE. Not just any exercise will work, mind you. But with exercise that elevates the heart rate to a point—thought to be about 60 to 75 percent of your heart rate maximum—your body creates a hormone in your bloodstream called BDNF (brain-derived neurotrophic factor). At that level of fairly intense exercise, your body does far more than build a strong cardiovascular system. It pumps significantly more oxygen and BDNF-laden blood into your brain. And that BDNF is not only the source of enhanced cognitive function but also the base ingredient for creating new brain cells.

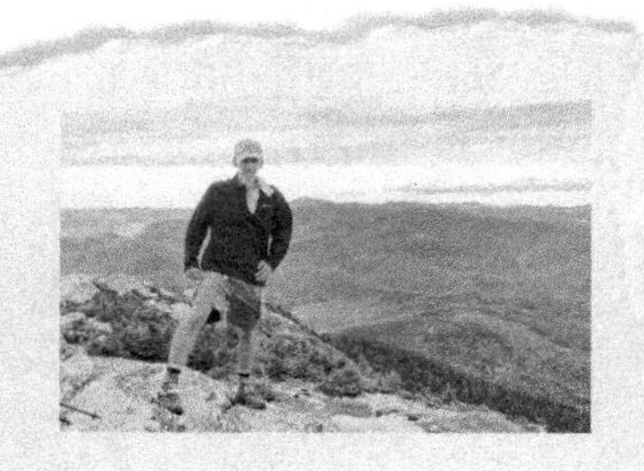

"I'm 63. I thru-hiked the Long Trail last year. I once thought of myself as more of a golfer than a hiker, but over the years, I became more interested in hiking. At first, my wife and I would do short hikes with the boys, and then I would do some longer solo hikes. I kind of got hooked on hiking around that time. It always feels great walking into the woods. I enjoy the challenge that hiking presents, the sights and smells of the forest, walking above treeline, the summits. I feel a sense of accomplishment after completing a difficult hike. I kick myself that I didn't start hiking in my teens and 20s instead of waiting until my 40s."

– Brian Cunningham, Massachusetts

Incidentally, this is the number one rationale for a

Fitbit or similar tracker with a heart rate monitor. You'll quickly learn how to get your body into the 60 to 75 percent zone, where you are doing the most good. How many steps you are taking is nice to know, but it's the quality of the steps that matter more. A day with 4,000 high-quality steps that elevate your heart rate is better than 8,000 slow, shuffling steps.

Now, it isn't quite as simple as just getting a heart rate tracker and getting your heart rate into the right zone, because as good as all that new BDNF will be for your brain, your brain needs to be cognitively stimulated to put that new BDNF to good use and build new neurons.

What kind of cognitive stimulation will do this? You need the kind of cognitive stimulation that involves using your brain to control and coordinate your body as it performs complex movements and fine motor skills. The more complex it is (involving the most muscles and high levels of exertion and mental processing), the better it is for your brain.

Can you guess where we're going with this?

As far as I can tell, the absolute best thing you can do to improve the function of your brain and to build new brain cells is hiking. This is pretty much why this book is trying to motivate you to get off the couch and start walking and exercising in such a way that you can then start hiking. Recall the 75-year-old gentleman I met trail running on Mount Washington? That man was a walking, talking BDNF factory.

Yes, there are other activities and exercises that will do this. But there is another concept that works in tandem with neurogenesis that we must understand to fully appreciate the amazing and unique benefits of hiking. That is the concept of neuroplasticity.

Neuroplasticity is the brain's ability to reorganize and rebuild itself by forming new neural connections or pathways. These neural pathways are the connections that link brain cells together. More neural pathways create a stronger, denser brain. And increased neural pathways are created through physical activity and learning.

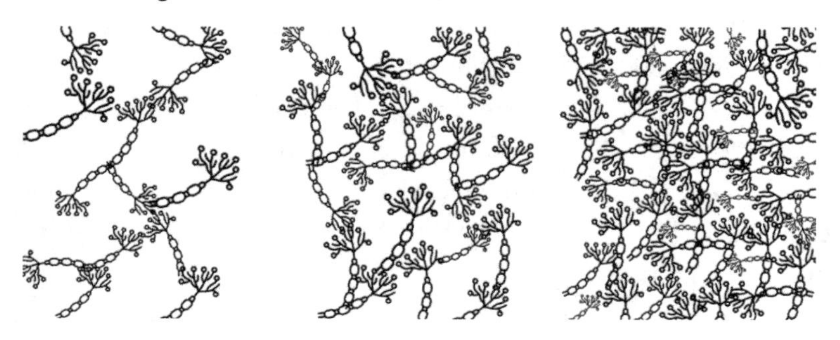

*Developing Denser Neural Pathways*

Learning to speak French creates more neural pathways in your brain, as does becoming an expert musician (piano playing seems to be exceptionally beneficial in this regard), and so does being expert at advanced mathematics. All these are good for creating extra neural pathways. However, none of these activities are as good as hiking, because they do not involve movement that elevates the heart rate in order to maximize the creation of BDNF. And none require the brain to coordinate repeated full-body, varied, complex movements. "An environment without exercise has little-to-no effect on neurogenesis," said Ryan Glatt, Psychometrist and Brain Health Coach at Pacific Neuroscience Institute.

Dementia, cognitive decline, Parkinson's, Alzheimer's are all among the biggest concerns the aging population has for the future. So, it makes complete sense that in structuring a fitness program, we must consider how it impacts the brain.

So, here's the important point: exercise isn't only about your body. Building muscles and conditioning your heart and circulatory system are important benefits, with many anti-aging properties, but I think of them as bonus side effects, because exercise is really about your brain.

## Perspective and Vision

There is another benefit to this kind of fitness: the natural vision improvement that comes from it, especially that which is acquired by being outdoors.

A number of complex small muscles control the eye. The eyeball itself is moved by six extraocular muscles, and the pupil is controlled by the tiny ciliary muscles attached to the pupil. These muscles focus the lens on an object by changing its shape as needed. If you are always indoors staring at a computer screen, those muscles do not get a chance to move much or use their full range of motion. When you stare at a screen for long periods, those muscles become strained and tense. That tension can actually diminish your eyesight.

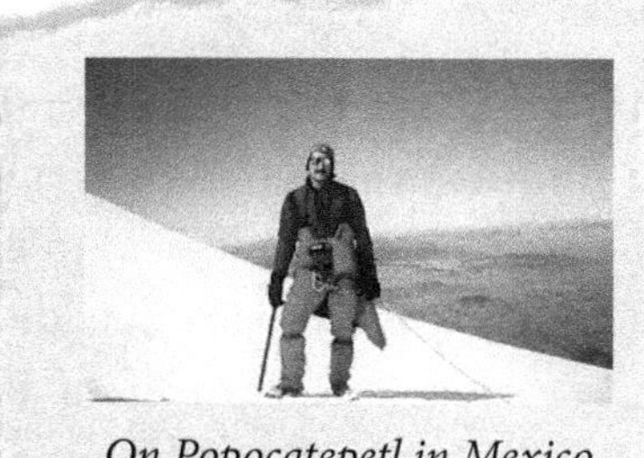

*On Popocatepetl in Mexico*

Perspective. Up high, above it all, I breathe better, I see better, I think better. I feel like I am part of something much bigger than myself, but also very humble and grateful. Being in a place like this, it becomes clear how small much of what you worry about really is in the grand scheme of things, and the stress melts away. It is not necessary to venture this high, or this far from home, to get this same perspective, to experience this feeling of awe that only getting outside can provide.

Think of it this way: if you sit still in a cramped airplane seat for a six-hour flight, your legs get tight and cramped up. When you deplane, your first steps are often stiff and awkward. Well, that's what happens to your eyes after days of staring at a screen.

By going outside frequently and looking at the world around you, your eyes are darting around and moving naturally to guide you through your movements. This needs to occur on a regular basis to keep those muscles flexible and in command of the full range of motion.

When you go outside, you look forward, outward, and up, not down and close. When you are outside, and you look to the horizon, your eyes focus to infinity. You use your depth perception abilities, and you see in three dimensions, not a flat-screen.

This enables the eye muscles to loosen up, remain flexible, and to use the full range of motion they are designed for. Failure to do this over a long period can result in slight changes in the shape of your eye and lead to diminished eyesight.

Also, when you are outside, your eyes perceive a more natural range of colors. Instead of the browns, greys, and unnatural colors of many indoor environments, being outside gives you all the greens and the blues. These natural outdoor colors are more soothing and thought to be better for your brain.

Some within the eye care industry are catching on to this. I got a note from my eye doctor recently with the following advice: "Reduce computer-related eyestrain—for every 20 minutes of screen time, look 20 feet in front of you for 20 seconds."

Your brain likes to be outside; it loves to be walking uphill, and it loves when you take your body on a hike. Put the brain first, and the body will follow.

# 14

# CAN'T I JUST JOIN A GYM?

*The fitness industry is one of the most profitable and persuasive businesses out there, but in terms of promised results, it has been a disappointing failure. There are very few fitness brands, technologies and commercial programs which actually deliver what they promise.*

— SINDHUJAA KUMAR IN *ENTREPRENEUR MAGAZINE*, 2018

The fitness industry boom of the last generation is not making us fitter as a population. The advent of large, corporate fitness companies, while useful places to get fit for some, also coincides with a massive obesity epidemic. So, something is out of whack. To some, fitness might even be considered a failed business model—in need of upgrades for an aging population. But there is hope for the fitness business if we re-engineer it.

I've been involved in the fitness industry since 1980—as a member, as an executive, and now as an entrepreneur trying to learn from its shortcomings to try to reinvent it. So, in this book about getting outside, I must first say: fitness clubs do have an important role in the fitness equation. But they need to do more. They need to focus more on outcomes. And gyms are not enough to get the kind of fitness I'm talking about here.

Sadly, to my way of looking at things, most gyms have too many shortcomings for too many people. The industry is still not delivering on its promise and potential, and it is still struggling to play a respected role in making the culture healthier and fitter.

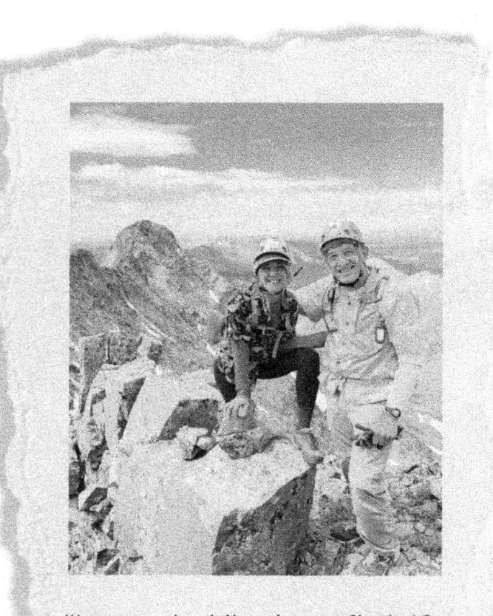

"I was not a hiker in my first 48 years. I was getting noticeably older and slower, and that motivated me to get in shape. A funny thing happened on the way to the mountain, the gym was nice, but the hikes were sublime–Just me, the woods and hills, and the miles. My secret weapon to get through stressful days at my office job are my lunchtime walks in the woods and thinking about past or future hiking experiences."

– Thorn Jarvis, Illinois

To some, the fitness industry is one of high-pressure sales, deceptive and unclear membership agreements, uncomfortable or intimidating membership experiences, predatory club employees, unclean, germy places, and more. So, while I am truly a fan of the fitness business, I am also a very harsh critic of it. It had, and still has, the potential to be the key linchpin in creating a fitter, healthier world. It should aspire to be the solution to the simmering, never-ending, and seemingly unsolvable healthcare crisis.

## Gyms and the Fitness Business

I was an insider in the gym/fitness world. Not only was I an active member of various fitness clubs, beginning around 1980, but I also was in senior management of the world's largest "big box" gyms at the time, Bally Total Fitness, which also owned Crunch Fitness.

I came to the fitness industry as an experienced marketer and consumer behavior expert. And even though I had been a participant in the fitness industry for 25 years—many of those years as a Bally member—I had never been behind the curtain or in a position to actually make changes. I was tasked with breathing new life into the company. It had become stagnant, membership numbers had leveled off, and the competition was intensifying.

So the first thing I did, rather than shoot blindly in the dark or listen to career insiders, was to dig deep behind the industry's somewhat insular way of looking at the business to study the major competitors and the up-and-comers (at the time this was 24 Hour Fitness, LA Fitness, Lifetime Fitness, Equinox, and Curves) to see what we could learn.

We launched over $1 million in consumer research on the industry, with particular emphasis on gaining insight about people who were not members and those who would never consider joining the big box gym world. We needed to know why. We talked to ex-members, we talked to members of competitive clubs, and we "mystery shopped" in all of them to experience membership for ourselves. Up to this point (2003), this kind of broad, deep, and objective consumer research had never been done in this industry.

What we learned was astounding at the time, but in retrospect, it was totally obvious:

1. **Many women were hesitant to join.** Or once they joined, they were hesitant or even afraid to go near "the cage," where the free weights were located, for fear of being ogled, harassed, or merely stared at by preening, leering, grunting weightlifters. Many said the same thing about our own employees.
2. **People felt they had to get fit *before* they joined a club,** or they'd be embarrassed, ridiculed, or judged. Fitness clubs, by their nature, tend to be very judgmental places, and members do scrutinize other members. It's a very body-centric environment, heightened by mirrors, locker rooms, and showers.
3. **People above age 50 were not comfortable** in the majority of gym environments. In addition to not liking the judgmental aspect, lack of cleanliness, and high noise levels, there was a deeply felt (though often hard to verbalize) desire to work out in a place where they were not massively outnumbered by all those pesky and much fitter younger people.

   The data bears this out. Ten years ago, fitness club membership plummeted as age increased. Up to age 45, membership percentage across all ages was about 30 percent. Over the age of 45, it went down to under 10 percent (Piper Jaffray Fitness Industry Report, 2014). This has improved a bit over the last decade—but more because of the older population's recognition that they absolutely must do something about their fitness, not because the industry consciously did much to be more welcoming.
4. **Many fitness club employees, and particularly personal trainers, had few of the skills essential to their chosen career.** They often were not caregivers but salesmen, and

not welcoming but arrogant and elitist. Instead of saying, "I know how to help you, and I care," they offered, "Look at my abs, don't you want to have abs like mine? See these biceps? I must know what I'm doing." Too many employees were not only incapable of guiding members to long-term results, but they were actually driving members away from the industry, perhaps forever.

5. **People complained about the music** because it's too loud. Often, gym members can't hear their own music in their headphones because it's polluted with the club's own 90-decibel sound system. Too many clubs operate on the narrow belief that members need that pounding music to get motivated.

As a result, the industry was not attracting the people who needed it most. It appealed to people who are already fairly fit, not insecure about their bodies, and not insecure about being vulnerable as a newbie in front of staring strangers. Some will gird up their courage and join anyway during the membership drives of December and January (lose weight in time for summer!). But they find it difficult to maintain a regular schedule, start missing workouts, and eventually let their membership lapse.

So, the industry does not attract all the people it could, and it does not retain as many members as it should. There's an extremely high degree of

> "I am going on 72. Have done all the 14,000-foot peaks in Colorado, many of them two, three, or four times. Still try to do a high one each year for my birthday. I keep hiking and working out in the gym. I work out every day early in the morning and hike most every weekend."
>
> – Ulli Limpitlaw, Colorado

churn: people join and quit, look for another club, join and quit again, buy a piece of home exercise equipment instead, and then stop using it because they are bored with it.

## Re-Engineering the Fitness Business

There is hope for the future of fitness, and many entrepreneurs are circling to fill the void, using both modern technology and a better understanding of human behavior to be more useful for more people. The fitness business is now finally starting to innovate rather than continue with a variation on the original big box theme. A few trends are described below.

**The Quantified Self movement** and the advent of Fitbit, Apple Watch, and numerous other activity and biometric tracking devices have engaged and invigorated the industry. Millions of individuals are now hyper-aware of the importance of activity, movement, and quality sleep. The measurement they permit does, indeed, provoke more activity. I believe this is only the start—data from these devices, tracking and collecting behavior, will increasingly be used to create more effective fitness programs.

**The medical fitness movement** is also very encouraging. Smart fitness entrepreneurs are starting to fill the space between the fitness business and the medical community by employing science-based exercise techniques and professional, customer-centric, results-oriented business practices. All of this is done with the dual objectives of:

1. Creating reciprocal relationships with the medical community, so doctors will readily prescribe fitness to their patients

2. Gaining subsidies and acknowledgment from the health insurance industry, who will recognize that fit, active people are far less expensive to insure than obese, inactive people.

**More professional personal trainers and coaches** are on the way. This is not just a matter of more certifications, but a shift toward trainers who have a science-based, results-oriented, caregiving mentality, rather than an aggressive sales and egocentric mentality. This new breed of trainers and coaches are attuned to the human behavioral aspects of motivating those who are unfit toward fitness. They are capable of building long-term, trusting relationships with their clients by focusing on positive outcomes.

Better yet, they work with clients to improve fitness beyond the gym. Exercises are designed to challenge both mind and body to improve different types of movement—strength, mobility, and balance. All are essential for living your life the way you want and will help prepare you to get outside.

**Small studios run by personal trainer owner/operators** will experience growth. The growth in this sector of the fitness business signals not only consumer dissatisfaction with some big box gym companies but also the desire for a personal human relationship with a personal trainer/coach who actually cares and puts your results and health as priority number one. All the technology in the world is not going to undo or suppress the need for these kinds of human interactions to motivate the unfit toward fitness.

Even with these future advances and the evolution within the gym business, we must recognize that even the best gym and the best trainer are not enough. To achieve the best kind of brain and body fitness results, we must transfer a portion of our fitness programs to the great outdoors. And the fitness industry should recognize this too and rather than see it as a competitive threat, embrace it.

Climber/hiker/trekker extraordinaire Josephine Johnson from Seattle (by way of New Zealand) would agree. This diminutive 61-year-old who radiates energy has honed her hiking and climbing skills step-by-step over two decades. And now, having climbed Mount Rainier, Kilimanjaro, and more, she gets it: "You can't get what I have in a gym. You've got to get out there."

So, yes, join a gym. Get a caregiver personal trainer if you can afford it. But recognize that a gym membership is not enough. To achieve full-body fitness, brain fitness, natural vision improvement, stress reduction, psyche-changing mental strength, and more, you must transfer a portion of your fitness program to the great outdoors.

And if you're a gym operator or a personal trainer, it would help your clients to offer programs that give them the skills and the fitness levels to be confident as they go outdoors. Getting fit in a gym and getting fit outside are not mutually exclusive. They work together very well.

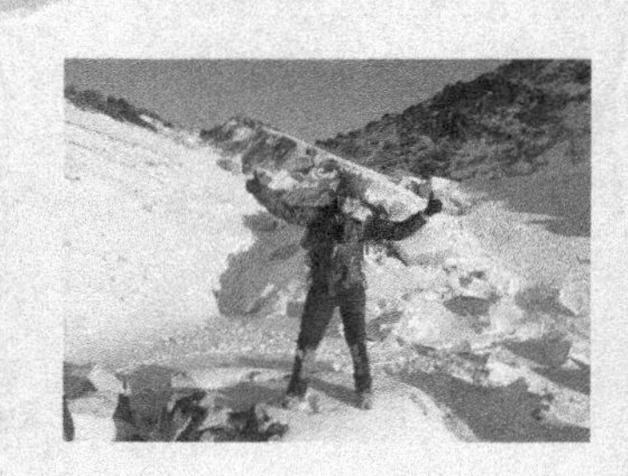

"I'm 62. I go to the mountains to find things, not lose things. I go to the mountains to widen my horizons, not narrow them. I go to the mountains not to escape what I leave behind, but to contemplate what I have. I go to the mountains for the sheer thrill of making my body move and to still my aching mind. If you are continually out there walking and moving, well, that's the best thing that you can be doing as a woman. Weight-bearing exercise staves off osteoporosis. It builds your skeletal frame. My doctor says she can't find anything wrong with me, and that I have the health of a 40-year-old, because of hiking."

– Josephine Johnson, Washington

*"Wholesome exercise in the free air, under the wide sky, is the best medicine for body and spirit."*

**– Sarah Louise Arnold**

SECTION 4

# Get Outside

# 15

# START WITH A WALK

*The way to get started is to quit talking and begin doing.*

— WALT DISNEY

What? A book about fitness, getting outside, and hiking that doesn't have specific advice until the last section? Well, by now, I'm sure you've figured out that this book is about more than hiking.

What we've been doing up to now has provided the context and the rationale for getting fit and doing it outdoors. We've delved into the demographics and implications of an aging, unfit, and inactive population, underserved by a fitness business that is not living up to its potential as a trusted part of the healthcare equation. We've reviewed the newest science of brain and body fitness and why it is so critical to understanding how this can be your pathway to living a happier, healthier, longer life.

As for the hiking part, I've been trying to ease you into it—to give you the many reasons why you should give this a try. And hopefully, you've been intrigued by my personal story and the stories and lessons that so many other hikers have accumulated and contributed along the way.

I'm aware that for some, the actual hiking part may be a bit of a hurdle. If that's you, this chapter will make it seem like a smaller hurdle. As with anything new, you have to start at the beginning and take those first small steps. If you're already a hiker or already have a fitness program, skim it fast and move on to the next chapter, where we talk about adding some hills.

What's important to recognize here is that you can attain a life-extending, health-improving, brain-enhancing level of fitness without staring at four walls in a sunless, breezeless spinning class or by watching the news on a gym treadmill with 90-decibel rap music pounding away, or by following along with a DVD in your basement four times a week.

Why not get the same physical benefits and much, much more by transferring a big part of your fitness efforts outside to nature's big, open, grassy, green, sunny, gymnasium and playground?

Before you begin, however: ***get a physical.*** If you've been inactive or have any concerns about your ability to walk or exercise, please see a physician before you start. You want to make sure your heart and cardiovascular system are not compromised; that your ankles, knees, and hips can take the strain; and that your balance is fine. Once you're cleared, your doctor should celebrate your desire to get fit in this manner.

## Getting Started Is Simple

Here's all you really need to begin:

**Comfortable walking shoes.** Proper footwear is the most important thing. Don't wear clogs, flip flops, or sandals. They will affect your gait, slow you down, introduce the possibility of blisters or other injuries, and they do not offer proper support for walking, exercising, or hiking. Sneakers or running shoes will do for starting out.

**If you smoke, quit.** Right now. Just do it. That goes for cannabis too. I just don't see anything that suggests either of those are part of living longer and better. You can get high on being outside much easier and cheaper. Plus, if you're going to quit these habits cold turkey, the perfect time to do it is when you begin a fitness program. Your entire body will thank you, and you'll really benefit from the extra lung power you get by quitting.

**Just start walking.** How simple is that? As we said earlier, it all begins with a single step. And that is true. But this is where we connect those single steps and start putting in some mileage.

**Get a fitness tracker.** This is something I feel pretty strongly about. The Quantified Self movement is incredibly useful. Fitbit, Garmin, Polar, Suunto, Apple Watch, and more. Take your pick. They are all fine. Measurement of your walks and hikes makes a big difference. It enables you to compare yourself to an earlier version of you, and thus, measure your progress. And tracking that progress (in steps, distance,

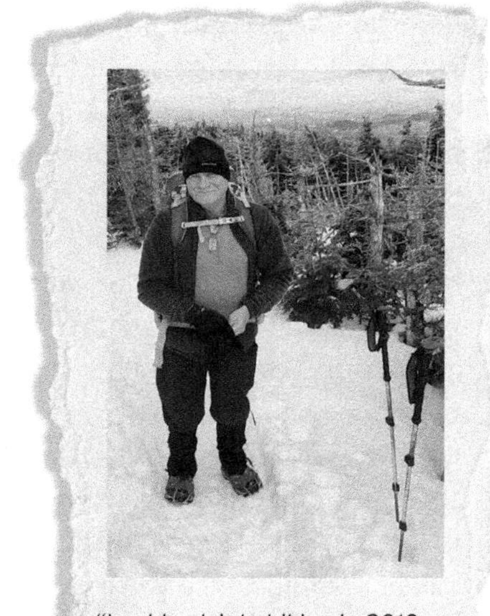

"I got back into hiking in 2010 when I was a couple of months shy of 61. I completed all 48 of the New Hampshire 4,000 footers in 2015 and finished the 67 New England 4,000 footers this August, just shy of my 70th birthday. I got back into hiking because a near-fatal auto accident in 2000 left me with severe leg injuries which require ongoing strenuous exercise to maintain my mobility."

– John Benham, New Hampshire

calories burned, flights climbed, etc.) is both motivational and fun. That's just for starters. As you progress, you're also going to want to carefully measure your heart rate, because a key element in a healthier brain and body is getting your heart rate elevated enough to trigger real physiological improvement.

## Walking Plus

The absolute best exercise for newbies is to get outside and take a brisk walk.

It's the most accessible and simplest exercise you can do. Throw in an occasional jog or sprint when you are able, and it is, without question, the best exercise for overall health and wellness. It has great aerobic benefits and also builds endurance and leg strength, which helps with core strength and overall balance. It boosts your energy level and immune system and has a minimal chance of leading to injury.

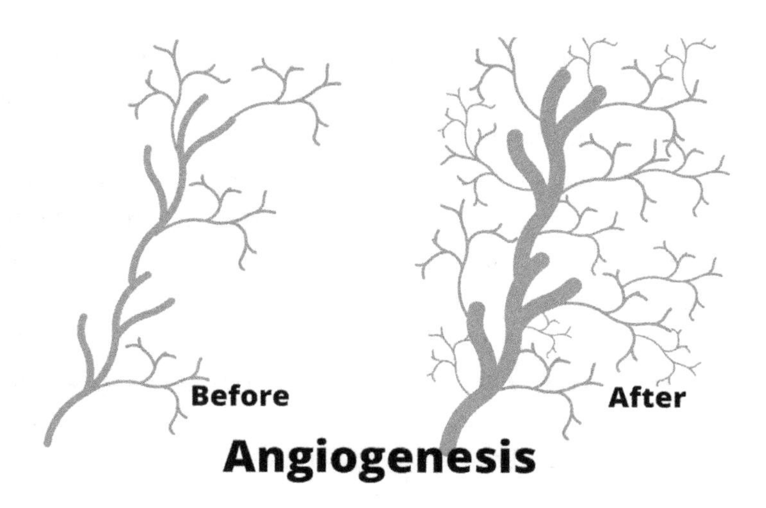


*Your body responds to exercise by growing a denser vascular system.*

Most likely, at some point soon, mere walking will not seem like enough exercise. When that happens, you can dial it up a bit. And you should make every effort to up the intensity because that is where the maximum benefits to brain health and longevity lie. Higher intensity exercise triggers angiogenesis (the growth of new, bigger blood vessels) and neurogenesis (the development of new brain cells and neural pathways). That's what this is all about. All that new circulation helps you develop stronger muscles, a stronger heart, and a sharper brain.

Once you get comfortable with your walking routine, you can quickly amp up the benefits by doing the following:

**Walk faster.** Pick up the pace. Give it a little more intensity, and you'll likely live longer as a result. Researchers at the University of Leicester report that fast walkers could live up to 15 years longer than people who move slowly. Our bodies have evolved to walk, and the more you do, and the faster you go, the better off you are (Fowler 2019).

And if your body tells you that you can go even faster, throw in a jog, or even a sprint at several points during any walk. The short boost to your heart rate that's triggered does wonders for helping you get to the next level.

**Walk farther.** More steps, more mileage, and more calories burned add up to more brain and body benefits. In a short amount of time, a two-mile walk will seem like your warmup, and you'll be adding distance effortlessly.

**Wear a pack.** Get a small backpack to carry the few items you'll need to make your longer walks comfortable. Throw in a couple of water bottles. Pack a rain jacket and umbrella. Throw in lunch, so you can make a whole day of it. A little extra weight on your back makes the legs work a little harder, causes your heart to beat a bit faster, and heightens the benefits to both brain and body. For what it's worth, I've been known to put 50–60lbs of gear in a big expedition backpack for a short, flat walk along the local bike path. I need to have that extra weight-bearing stress on the system, so I feel like I'm really working out.

**Wear ankle weights.** Ankle weights are controversial for some fitness trainers because if they are used wrong while running, or if they are too heavy, they can stress joints, tendons, or ligaments to the point of injury. It's best to limit them to no more than two pounds on each leg to start, and only use them while walking—never while running.

I've been using them for a long time. Sometimes I leave them on all day, throughout my regular day-to-day at the office, and I've never had any problems with knees or ankles from them. I like the idea that the ankle weights make my sneakers and trail shoes feel like climbing boots (which is great preparation for an actual climb). So, give them a try to boost your workout. But if they cause you inordinate soreness, they might not be for you.

**Walk on the beach.** The texture and instability of sand make it an exceptionally good boost in the degree of difficulty, especially for your calves and ankles. Have you ever noticed the ankles and calves of a beach volleyball player? It's the sand that does that. A three-mile hike in the sand feels like double that to your calves.

**Walk uphill.** Nothing beats walking uphill, as far as I'm concerned. And that is because of the extra exertion it requires. You are fighting gravity to move the weight of your body with every step. It engages muscles in your legs and hips that are hardly ever activated on flat ground. The result is an elevated heart rate.

**Use Nordic poles.** These are essentially ski poles with a protective and grippy rubber tip. Using them helps burn more calories and works more muscles than conventional walking. It is a non-snow version of Nordic skiing. You use your arms to get a little extra propulsion as you walk, and in the process, you work parts of your upper body, giving you an elevated heart rate and a more intense cardiovascular workout.

And if you have balance issues, using Nordic poles gives you two more points of contact with the ground, thus helping prevent falls. In fact, many physical therapists are recommending Nordic poles instead of walkers for some rehab patients because they promote more natural posture. Premature use of a walker can actually accelerate further declines in both balance and gait. Groups using Nordic poles are popping up all over the country, and it should not be hard to find a good pair of poles and a nice group to join.

**Take the stairs.** I have a saying: "I always take the stairs, so I can always keep taking the stairs." If you work in an office building, shop at a mall, park in a parking garage, live in an apartment building, etc. there is often the option of elevator, escalator, or stairs. Unless it's completely impractical to do so, I always use the stairs, even

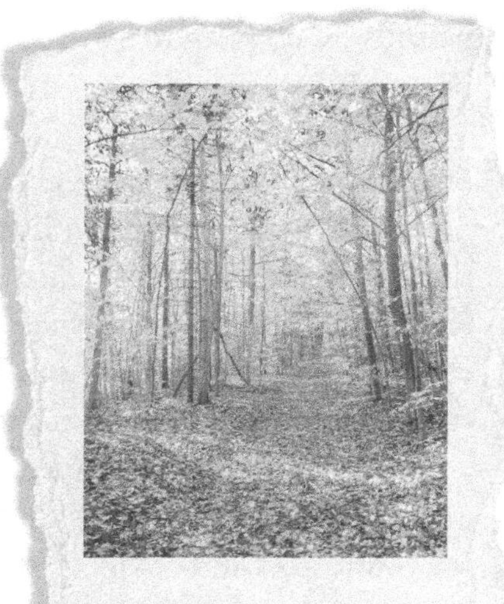

**Easy Trails**

An easy trail will be flat or only slightly uphill with minimal obstacles. Despite the relative ease of these trails, they reduce stress, soothe the spirit through sensory stimulation, and benefit both brain and body with exercise. Places like this are very accessible almost everywhere, and they contain immense rewards if you are able to walk away from the hustle and bustle of civilization, even if only for a few hours.

with luggage. I'm quite disciplined about this (likely because stair climbing is possibly my core competence in this world!). You'll be surprised how easy it is to do and how much good it will do you.

All these things increase the intensity of your walk, raise your heart rate, work your muscles a bit more, and put the right kind of stress on weight-bearing muscles and bones.

Once you decide to start walking and set your intensity, know that walking outside—especially on a trail—is exponentially better for your brain and your body and significantly more cognitively stimulating than any indoor experience on a treadmill or exercycle.

## Strategies to Keep at It

Even the best of plans can get derailed at times—life happens. But there are some things you can do to help ensure you stick to your new program:

**Keep it simple.** If you haven't had an exercise routine before, the simpler it is when you start, the more likely you'll be to stick with it. You can add more later once you make this a habit. It will eventually get too easy, and that's when it's time to add something extra or new.

**Keep it realistic.** When you're starting, don't set goals that are too far out there or too hard. Your comfort zone can only stretch so far at first, or the fear takes over, and you regress or quit. Don't expect overnight results.

**Use that tracker.** Measure yourself via Fitbit, Apple Watch, or another device. But don't weigh yourself. I've found that single-mindedness about weight is the worst way to track progress. Bodyweight doesn't always respond immediately, and it is not the best measure of your fitness level. When weight is the focus, and it doesn't drop quickly, the result is often a decrease in motivation. Steps, time, and how you feel are better metrics at first. Relax. The weight will come off in time.

**Find some friends or join a group.** Nordic walking groups are a good example. The feeling of responsibility when you know a friend is waiting, the motivation of peer pressure, and the social aspect of exercising with a group can be very helpful for staying on track.

**Give it time.** It can take 40 to 60 days to instill a new habit into your brain. Remind yourself that you are doing this for your brain, for your family, and for you.

Far too many people are house-bound, office-bound, city-bound, or gym-bound. We need to find more time to exercise outside in a natural setting—ideally, far away from the hustle and bustle of civilization. Starting with a walking program is a simple way to break out of your old habits, set yourself off in the right direction, and prepare for even more vigorous and beneficial activities.

---

*"Exercising both body and brain can help people stay healthier longer. The new thinking about aging considers not just how long one lives, but how vibrant one stays later in life."*

– **Outside Magazine**, *January 2020*

---

# 16

# HEAD FOR THE HILLS

*Research shows that hiking has a positive impact on combating the symptoms of stress and anxiety.*

– GREGORY A. MILLER, PH.D., PRESIDENT OF THE AMERICAN HIKING SOCIETY

More and more, people are looking for a new option for fitness. Bored with their gym workouts, mobile apps, and home exercise equipment, they're ready for the physical and cognitive benefits delivered by getting outside.

And more and more companies and organizations are capitalizing on this shift, using their marketing efforts to entice people to get outside. REI's entire business model focuses on helping people "Get Outside," and their #OptOutside program encourages employees and customers to skip the Black Friday shopping madness and go outdoors instead. Similarly, *Outside Magazine's* mission is "To inspire active participation in the world outside …" and L.L. Bean advises its patrons to "Be an Outsider."

Practically every ad for senior-living facilities or adult communities has visuals of their residents happily forest bathing and hiking. Outdoor recreation and equipment are currently among the fastest-growing segments of the economy, contributing $778 billion to total US gross output plus 5.2 million jobs (Arvesen 2019). Even *Time* magazine has written on the trend, noting that hiking is "the perfect mind-body workout" (Heid 2017).

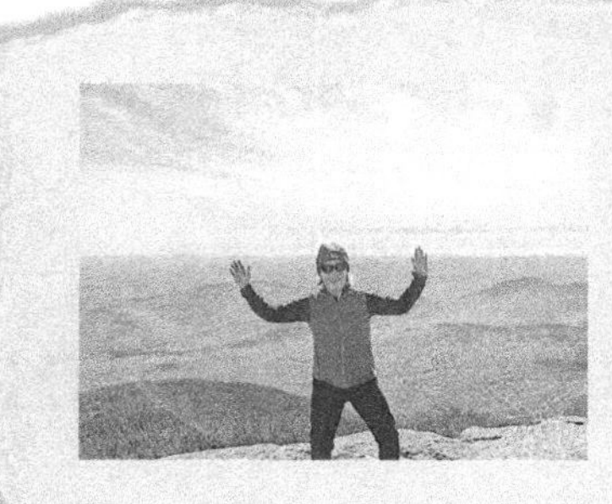

"We began first with smaller local hikes to get familiar with the area, and then after 15+ hikes, we were ready to try a new challenge—a winter hike in the Whites. We snowshoed Mt. Willard and were hooked by the incredible views. The feeling we got from our time in the woods was so recharging that our hikes compelled a 'clear-the-calendar, must do' priority. Nothing else has ever given me the enormous sense of well-being and confidence boosting that I get from hiking. One day on Mt. Pierce, with freezing rain drizzling down and embracing it all, was the beginning of our commitment to do all 48 of the New Hampshire 4,000 footers—in less than two and one-half years. We completed our quest, and I've never felt in as good physical shape as I do now."

– Cathy Carabello,
New Hampshire

## The Steps You Take

If you've been using a fitness tracker, you might know that you take about two thousand steps per mile. That information is a good starting point, but it's important to know that not every step is equal in terms of what it's doing for your fitness.

The majority of the walking we do (the steps we take during the course of a day or even those on a treadmill) is done on autopilot. You really don't think very much about those steps, and it's better than being sedentary. But it's not nearly as beneficial as the steps you take outside. When you are hiking, you must switch off the autopilot and pay attention to every step. As a result, the very nature of hiking—walking uphill over uneven and unpredictable ground—is an intense brain and body workout that is ideal for building new neural pathways, great leg strength, increased heart strength, and more.

## What to Take

For me, the difference between walking and hiking is that hiking requires a backpack. When you're going further afield, a few miles and hours from your car at the trailhead, you'll need a few things to make the trip safer and more pleasant.

I was a Boy Scout, so "Be prepared" is foremost in my mind here. Let me assure you that the equipment you need for most hikes is very minimal:

- A comfortable pair of hiking boots with ankle support
- A small backpack
- Water bottle(s)
- Rain protection
- Sun protection
- Pocket knife
- Compass and whistle
- Headlamp or flashlight
- Basic repair kit (duct tape!)
- Basic first aid kit
- Extra pair of socks

Of course, bring your cell phone too. But don't be dependent on it, because the signal often fades on a trail, it runs out of power, and water kills it instantly.

I'll wager that if you're not a hiker yet, you'll be thinking "repair kit, compass, whistle, pocketknife? Extra socks? I don't need that stuff." You probably won't, but in the spirit of "Be Prepared," go to GetOutside.online, and I'll explain why you do. For now, let's just say that the list above, which weighs 10 pounds at most, can mitigate 99 percent of the situations that can change a simple day hike into an uncomfortable, miserable, or even dangerous experience.

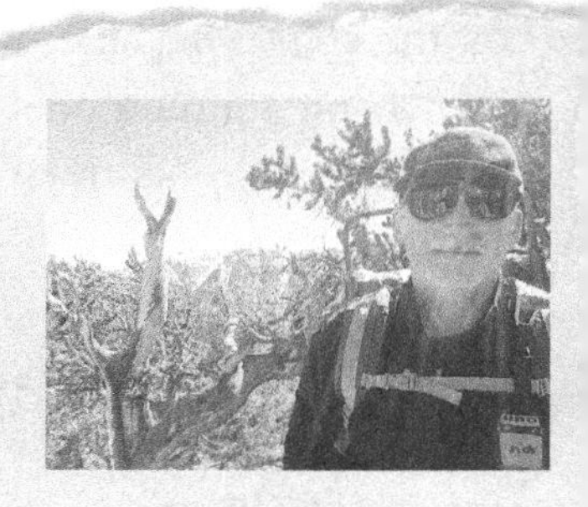

*Mount Charleston, Nevada one hour from the Las Vegas Strip*

People tell me all the time how they don't have anywhere to hike. I hear: I live in the city; it's so hard to get outside; there are no decent places for outdoor exercise; and so on. You'd be amazed at how accessible the outdoors and wilderness can be. For instance, here I am on Mount Charleston, only one hour northwest of the Las Vegas Strip. A few hours up the trail, it's another world—well-kept trails, big mountains, real wilderness, snow year-round, altitude, and wide vistas. The same goes for Mount Baldy, which is close to Los Angeles. Simple little micro-adventures like these pay big dividends in the mental and physical return on investment.

## Start with Short Hikes

Wherever you live, there will be places only a short drive away where you can put on your backpack and escape from your routine with a short hike.

Do this: Type "hikes near me" into your favorite search engine, and you'll be opening up a world of opportunities for short hikes that can get you started. Almost every part of the country has "Rails-to-Trails" locations, organized by a nonprofit organization dedicated to creating and promoting the nationwide network of walking and hiking trails that are made from former rail lines. These tend to be flat and pretty tame, though often beautiful, and it's hard to imagine a better resource for the beginner looking for places to start.

Once you start looking for options, you'll see numerous opportunities to get outside, put on the backpack, and start walking. Short hikes of two or three miles, an hour or two at most, are all you need to begin. And you might be surprised at where this can lead.

My trekking friends from Melbourne, Australia, Jim and Jenny Swinden, are a perfect example of how you can start small and work your way up in increments over time to a demanding high-altitude trek.

"We live on the beach, and it all started by doing 7-kilometer walks, run right here at home, on flat ground," says Jim. "It was an incremental thing. We started with little walks and hikes and experimented. It's become a big thing for us now," according to Jenny.

They graduated to hiking the Cumberland Way across the Lake District in England and then to the Camino Real in Spain. And with a combination of training and hiking, they advanced to the very rugged high-altitude Everest trek.

These are fantastic accomplishments. Only a generation ago, they were considered undoable over the age of 60 by many so-called fitness experts. But anti-agers like Jim and Jenny have helped raise the bar higher. As we have seen in the stories throughout the book, many hikers see themselves as ageless, and slowing down is not on the agenda.

In fact, I saw Jim and Jenny accomplish something that a generation ago would have been considered extreme and foolishly excessive. The last day of the Everest trek is a very rugged 15-mile day of downhill, uphill, downhill, with a final five-mile uphill grind.

That particular day, the weather did not cooperate, and they were forced to walk that very challenging trail in a typhoon. They endured a heavy, driving rain for hours, with bone-chilling wind, minimal visibility, thunder, and lightning. Given a choice, no sane person would have done it. But there really was no choice. The plane was leaving the next morning and missing it would have caused many days of delay. So, they called on all their reserves, experience, and training, and just did it. There was no drama or real danger because they'd worked their way up over time to have the confidence and ability to make it possible.

What do they have in common with a newbie, about to consider going down a similar path? They began by walking. And they progressed to short hikes, then longer hikes, and then to world-class treks.

Not everyone will want to take it that far. But you can garner the same benefits to brain and body and the same gains to health and longevity with smaller hikes, closer to home. And you'll never know how far you can take it until you begin.

## Speaking of Rain

Can you hike in the rain? Should you hike in the rain? Yes, absolutely.

The most intense sensory experience I've ever had in my many, many years of hiking came on a short, two-mile walk into The Flume Gorge in New Hampshire in heavy rainfall.

Flume Gorge is a narrow ravine, about sixty feet deep and a quarter of a mile long, carved through solid rock by meltwater from the mountains above it. It contains a couple of waterfalls and a raging stream that continues to do the carving. Just as I arrived, the rain became very intense—driving, heavy, and thick. And as

I walked into the entrance of the gorge, thunder and lightning were suddenly concentrated right above me. The waterfall and the stream intensified and magnified the rain and thunder echoing in the canyon. The sound bounced from side to side, again and again. I had anticipated this might be interesting in the rain, so in addition to my rain suit, I had also brought an umbrella to make sure I could enjoy it to the fullest.

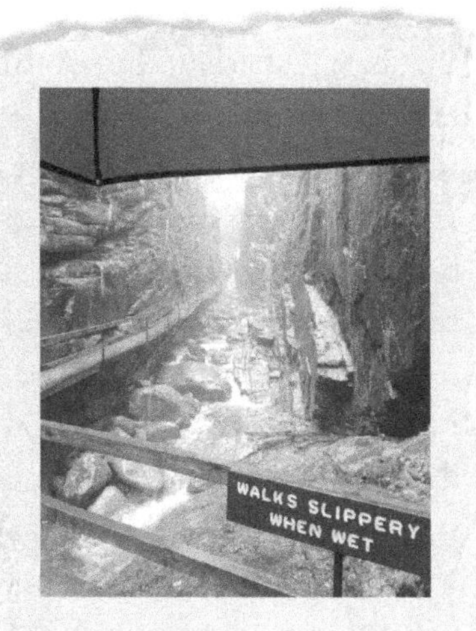


*The Flume Gorge, New Hampshire*

One of the most memorable and intense moments of my 50 years of hiking was the hour I spent under an umbrella soaking in the intensity of a multi-sensory driving thunderstorm and hailstorm at the Flume Gorge in New Hampshire. An easy 30 minutes from the parking lot, it is a whole world away. I often recall this experience as a way to invoke focus, calm, and heightened mindfulness.

I'm glad I did because the experience was exponentially greater than anything I had anticipated. I was able to stand in the center of The Flume, just feet from the torrent, with its vertical walls 10 feet on either side of me and enjoy this experience for about 45 minutes. It was an overwhelming, nonstop sensory assault—the sound and fury of nature at its best. The energy I absorbed was palpable, real, powerful, and invigorating. And oh my, what an incredible mindfulness session!

A sensory experience like that isn't just about the soothing and invigorating sound of rain. It's also biochemical. It's petrichor—the scent you breathe in when it rains, the result of water droplets falling on dry leaves and ground. Falling rain clears the air of dust, pollen, and microbes, so you breathe in better air, laden with petrichor, the scent of nature.

I've felt versions of this before, but this one experience was at a whole new level, and it reminded me that while it's sometimes tempting to skip a hike or walk because it's raining, you never know what you might be missing.

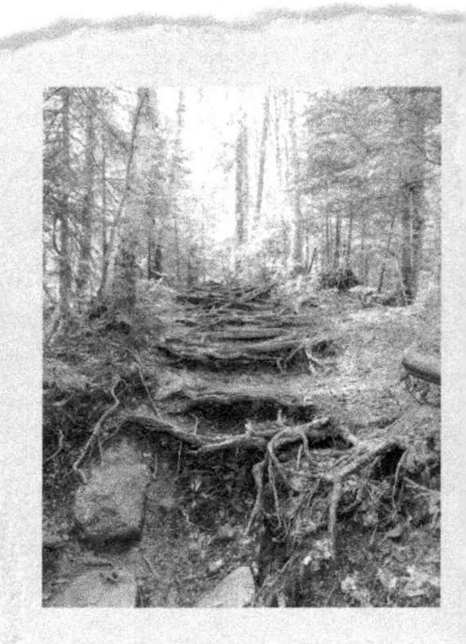

**Medium Trails**

Medium difficulty trails add challenges but also benefits. Steeper and more rugged, uneven and unpredictable, riddled with rocks and roots, they require vigilance, extra endurance, and leg strength, plus a level of confidence you gain from experience on easier trails. But the higher intensity works the brain and the body in ways you cannot get on a treadmill or a Stairmaster in the gym. The calorie burn is high, but the main benefits are the fountain-of-youth type benefits you start to feel from the boost to blood flow and oxygen surging through your body and brain.

## Getting Uphill

Now, if you're thinking that getting outside involves exotic trips to Colorado, the Alps, or mountain peaks of any sort, I want to assure you that's not the case. Pretty much wherever you go, there will be a source of untamed natural wilderness that's not too far away. And it's even true close to large cities like Los Angeles, New York, and Las Vegas.

Those are probably not the first places you think of when considering hiking options. But outside options are surprisingly accessible in many major metropolitan areas, and they present an interesting juxtaposition between city and wilderness.

There is powerful magic in the remote, high, wild places, and they can get into your head in a big way because the experience is so multifaceted and multisensory. That's where you can find those exponential benefits of being outside.

And you only have to get just a little bit off the beaten path to find places where there are no car horns, trucks rumbling, brakes screeching, phones ringing, background conversations, or someone else's bad music blaring loudly. Instead, you hear the wind, rustling leaves, birdsongs, your own footsteps, and your own heightened breathing. With every exhalation, you feel the stress evaporating, fading more and more into the background.

Then there are the vistas. You'll behold a panorama of color and shape in every direction and feel both powerful and small at the same time. And your eyes, which are usually accustomed to only looking across a room, at a computer screen, or just gazing small distances, can focus into infinity. Taking it all in relaxes eye muscles and opens the senses so rapidly, you can practically feel your brain saying, "Thank you."

And of course, there's the exertion. The accelerated heart rate and fatigue that result from getting to a remote or high place light up your now grateful brain like nothing else. You're pumping such amazing amounts of extra oxygen and blood through your head, that you are actually growing new brain cells in addition to strengthening your musculature and burning excess fat.

And, as if the physiological effect isn't enough, there's also an incredible psychological effect. The higher and farther you roam and the harder it is to get to a place, the more confident you become. You gain a sense of accomplishment that you can only feel if you've done it yourself.

This is very potent alchemy. But it's the contrast between the wild places and the daily grind most of us endure that really interests me. On the one hand, you have concrete, steel, pavement, technology, and all the cacophony and man-made trappings of civilization. On the other hand, there is solitude, granite, glaciers, snow, spruce, and pine—much of it pristine, unchanged for millennia, and untouched by civilization. The contrast is wonderful.

Going back and forth between these two worlds is mind-expanding. In the city, most of your movements are on flat, uniform ground, and your mind barely gives walking a thought. There is minimal risk. In the mountains, movement is rarely on level ground, and nearly every single step requires focus, concentration, effort, and balance on uneven, unforgiving, 100-percent-natural terrain—where occasionally a misstep can lead to serious injury or death. One world is set up to be safe and predictable. The other is primitive, wild, and unforgiving.

The stark contrast between city and wilderness, sometimes less than half a day apart, is a curious thing. I think it's like speaking two languages, forcing your brain to switch back and forth to adapt as needed. It definitely expands and broadens your perspective.

The best part is that all the above is transferable. You come back from these adventures, alternating between wilderness and city, as an enhanced version of yourself. You are more capable, more energetic, more creative, more relaxed, more focused, more self-assured, and more of whatever you need in order to accomplish great things in your career and your life.

And it's addictive. This is why those of us who go up into the wild go back again and again.

If you do not know this particular sensation, why not give it a try? It doesn't have to be a remote, frigid peak in a far-off land. There's almost always a way to replicate this experience on a small scale to get an inkling of the full effect. Start small—an uphill walk to a vista on a sunny day. Pick a location that's far enough away to require some effort and heavy breathing and is one that will get you to a place away from crowds, cell phones, and cars. There, you can look out at the world from a different perspective—both literally and figuratively. You just might get hooked.

---

*"You're off to great places, today is your day. Your mountain is waiting, so get on your way."*

**– Dr. Seuss**

---

# 17

# GET HIGHER

*We are designed to be wild, and by living tamely we make ourselves sick and unhappy.*

—DR. JOHN RATEY

At this point, we're going to assume you're ready to hike a little further from home, a little deeper into the woods, a little higher into the mountains. That's going to require some new skills in addition to extra fitness and sound judgment.

The more remote places are both breathtakingly beautiful and dispassionately unforgiving. They do not care if you're not physically ready for their challenges. So, it is important to go there with as much preparation as you can manage. Not only does it make for a more enjoyable adventure and reduce the potential for injury, but it also can be a lifesaver. The fitter you are, the better you can adapt to the unexpected—a fall, bad weather, getting lost, darkness, avalanche, etc.—and the more likely you will be able to overcome any obstacles in your path.

## New Skills You Need

**Learn how to read a map.** Virtually every designated hiking location has a free trail map available online—free and downloadable. Often, they are in a box at the start of the trail. There really are no acceptable excuses for not having a map of the area you plan to explore.

I recommend getting it a few days beforehand and studying it. With just 15 minutes of research, you can not only get the maps you need but also find reviews and route descriptions of nearly every trail on planet earth. You need to develop a basic sense of north, south, east, and west, and it's also extremely helpful to know what time sunset is, and you need to have an idea of the weather forecast.

Of course, you could use the many ubiquitous smartphone apps for navigation and route descriptions. Some are quite good. I use AllTrails, Gaia, and 3D Maps, but there are many others. You'll need to familiarize yourself with how they work before you need them, though. Try them out on a neighborhood walk.

It's important to remember that due to weak cell signals in many of these off-road locations and the shortened battery life that mapping apps cause, it's best not to be solely dependent on technology for finding your direction. It's shocking to me how many people each year become totally disoriented on a trail, only a mile or two from their car, and only feet away from an easy trail. This can result in costly, manpower-intensive search and rescue efforts, or spending an uncomfortable, cold night sitting on a log, waiting for sunrise.

Seriously, you should not venture out alone if your directional skills are poor, or if you cannot read a map and use a compass. If you're uncomfortable with map reading and want to learn more, there are plenty of classes—not only online, but also at most outdoor shops.

**Research your hike in advance.** In short, have a plan. In addition to familiarizing yourself with the map, you should also make an estimate of how long it will take to do this walk or hike and confirm what time sunset will be. Establish what time you're leaving and what time you expect to be back. And give yourself a cushion to be sure you finish before sunset unless you are totally prepared and don't mind walking in the dark. If it's a relatively flat hike, a pace of 20 to 30 minutes per mile is a good guess. If it's steeper, figure 30 to 60 minutes per mile. Proper planning of your hike also includes letting someone else know your plans, such as friends, family, and often the nearby ranger. Then check in with them when you are done.

**Check the weather.** This is so obvious, yet so frequently ignored. Read the weather forecast to make sure you're prepared. This should influence what clothing, equipment, and route you choose. Think about how you'll stay dry if you get caught in rain or snow or whether you need to postpone due to inclement conditions.

**Water and food.** Nothing makes me shake my head more than coming across an unprepared hiker, still heading uphill in the late afternoon, many miles off the beaten path, with no pack, no hat, the wrong shoes, no headlamp, etc. But the part that gets me the most is when they are also carrying a small water bottle. Nothing says, "I'm out of my element" more than a person five miles from the trailhead, sun going down, no backpack, carrying a single plastic bottle of water in their hand.

**Don't be that person.** You are risking discomfort and injury to yourself and to the rescue crew that may have to come to get you in the middle of the night. I can't stress it enough: Make sure you are carrying the basic equipment items you might need if you are heading into the hills. **But most importantly, make sure you have enough water.**

## A Few Extras I've Learned Through the Years

As much as I'm advocating that getting outside provides a better type of fitness than you can get in a gym, I am not anti-gym at all. It's not enough for complete brain and body health in my view, but it's an integral part of the equation. Fitness gained during gym time provides the extra boost needed to complete more demanding adventures and be safe while doing them. So, I do try to get in a couple of gym visits a week.

When I work out at a gym, I focus on:

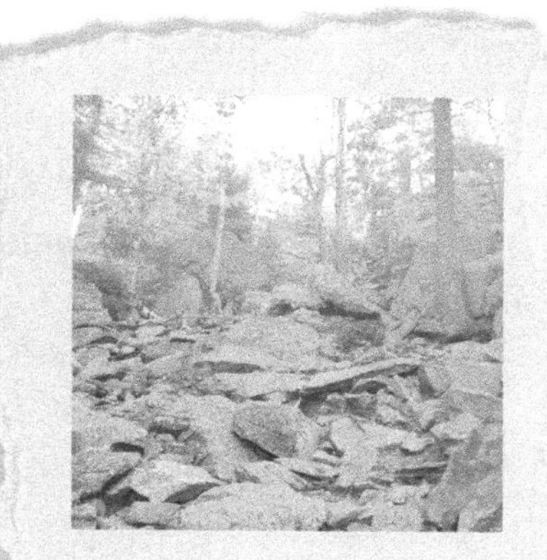

*Difficult Rocky Trail*

**Hard Trails**

Hard trails like this are yet another degree higher in both difficulty and benefits. Steeper and even more rugged, they demand greater endurance, balance, and leg strength that can be developed by mastering medium difficulty trails.

But the benefits: every step you take, up or down, requires your eyes and your brain to control and continually recalculate complex patterns of movement involving many muscles. It's an exceptional cardiovascular workout and a powerful brain workout that can trigger neurogenesis—the creation of new neural pathways—which builds cognitive reserves that can protect you from cognitive decline.

1. **Squats.** I do massive amounts of squats, all variations, with both free weights and leg-press machines.
2. **Toe raises.** It's such a simple exercise, and you can do it anywhere. Having fit ankles, feet, and calves are crucial for walking and hiking, so you cannot do too many of these.
3. **Box Jumps.** Up and down. You need to have a little plyometric (explosive) muscle power, so jumping up and jumping down, even 6 or 12 inches, can get you started and has big benefits.
4. **Lunges.** I do all kinds, both with and without weights, to keep the hips strong, loose, and flexible.
5. **Push-Ups.** They're such a basic move, yet they work the chest, shoulder, arm, and core muscles.

I often do a lot more than this, but the five moves above cover the basics and are good skills to build. Remember, you don't have to master them all at the start. But do start—begin where you are and work up to them. But, fitting in some workout time at home or at the gym is important. You need to have a little fitness edge that will enable you to hike longer and faster. And that will open up the possibility of so many more interesting and exciting hikes, climbs, and adventures.

In addition to basic fitness training, beginning hikers should get comfortable with easy three-to-five-mile hikes in the woods. That's a pretty good starting point to understand what your abilities are, and then you can take it from there. It's not uncommon to progress to the point where you can do ten miles or more of rugged hiking. That's a superb goal to shoot for.

Frankly, it's not uncommon these days for hyper-fit hikers to do double that on a regular basis, but since it's not a competition, we're not going to dwell on those extremes. You should hike your own hike—no need to compare yourself to anybody else. Compare yourself to you, and step by step if you apply yourself, you will improve.

## Taking it to the Next Level

When I'm preparing for a bigger adventure, I pack in as much local uphill time as I can (on smaller micro-adventures). If I'm going for a multi-day excursion to New Hampshire or Colorado, I put in as much time as possible beforehand in the local Connecticut hills, getting as much uphill mileage as I can, while carrying an extra-heavy pack.

For multi-day backpacking trips, it's important to make sure you work your legs hard on consecutive days to fully prepare. If I'm going on an extensive international trek or climb, I do all that, plus, in the 60 days beforehand, I add as much time on smaller mountains as I can fit into my schedule.

For years, Mount Washington in New Hampshire has been my training ground for the higher peaks of the Seven Summits. Mount Rainier was my training ground for the bigger peaks in North and South America, which in turn, were preparation for Antarctica and Nepal.

I'm not a natural runner, so I don't do much distance running. I prefer short jogs with occasional sprints thrown in. I love the up-and-down variations in heart rate that result from a sprint, walk, sprint, walk, run, walk, sprint training. And I often do it with a pack on my back. It increases the training effect, and it also reminds me of what I'm training for—hiking and climbing—which I like to keep in mind as motivation.

So, here's what I do year-round: I try to get out at least a couple of times a week. Sometimes it's a good hike; sometimes it's a simple walk/jog through the nearby reservoir. Sometimes it's back and forth in my driveway with a backpack and/or ankle weights. When I travel for business, sometimes it's walking up and down in the stairwell of the hotel. Thirty minutes of that, as boring as it sounds, is infinitely more doable and beneficial than 30 minutes on a treadmill at the gym.

I also often deliberately overpack, making my pack heavier than it needs to be. I'm not in a race, so there's no need to emphasize speed, and I do like to be over-prepared. I also don't like to be dehydrated. I consume a lot of fluids, so I usually pack at least 3 liters of water for a day out.

I'm not much of a fan of ultra-light hiking because I think it leaves you vulnerable, and as I get older, I don't really want that kind of risk. I carry extra gear and my first aid kit. I always have a change of clothes, extra socks, warmer clothing than I need, and a lightweight emergency blanket.

I also carry a GPS device for emergencies, and I carry at least one, (sometimes two) battery chargers for my phone. Every time you read about a hiker rescue in the paper, the culprit is almost always a cell phone that ran out of power. An eight-ounce battery charger eliminates that risk entirely.

Sometimes I bring binoculars, and sometimes I carry more than my phone for photography. Even for a day hike, I make sure I've got a headlamp. Dusk can sneak up on you, and a headlamp is a pretty lightweight insurance policy against being lost in the dark. I'm not suggesting the ultralight equipment philosophy is wrong; it's just not for me. The older I get, the more I prefer to be prepared for the worst-case scenario.

There's an old saying in hiking and climbing: "How can my pack be so heavy? It's filled with stuff that doesn't weigh anything at all." That may be true, but that "stuff" adds up, and you have to be the judge of what works for you. By the time you get to some more advanced hiking, you'll have enough of your own experience and judgment to gauge what you need and how much you're comfortable carrying.

Finally, several days before a bigger adventure, I recommend my favorite type of training hike. This should only be done when you have a good sense of your abilities, but it goes like this: Put on a heavy pack and head off into the hills. Walk as far as you possibly can, until you cannot take another step. Take a break and then walk a mile or two further. And then, when you really can't take another step, realize that you are many miles from your car, and you have a clear choice—lie down in the woods and freeze to death, or find the energy and the willpower to turn around and head back home.

You don't want to do this training exercise until you're sure you can handle it. But trust me, it makes you confident in your abilities, and gets you to the next level.

---

*"I love the mountains passionately. I have signed a sort of contract with them. And in them I will live out my life. Mountains are where nature offers her most beautiful contrasts. Nature offers the mountains to me, and I have consecrated my life to them. Without them, I would feel condemned to death."*

– **Walter Bonatti**, legendary mountaineer

---

# 18

# THE CRUCIBLE OF THE MOUNTAINS

*We who go mountain-scrambling know that each height, each step, must be gained by patient, laborious toil, and that wishing cannot take the place of working; that many a difficulty must be encountered, and many an obstacle must be grappled with, or turned, but we know that where there's a will, there's a way; and we come back to our daily occupations better fitted to fight the battle of life, and to overcome the impediments which obstruct our paths.*

— EDWARD WHYMPER, FIRST MAN ATOP THE MATTERHORN

Does anyone actually have an obstacle-free existence? Of course not. So, it makes sense to see your life as a never-ending series of lessons to be learned, with difficulties, hurdles, and trials that you must overcome. Doesn't it always seem as though every time you get past a tough period, just when you think you're in the clear for a while, some new challenge pops up, with a new test?

And that's the thing I like the most about hiking and climbing—they are wonderful analogies and the perfect preparation for the modern lives we lead and the challenges we face. They can prepare us and teach us how to confront and overcome these situations.

Most people do eventually reach a breaking point, either physical or mental, when faced with too many challenges. For most, though, that breaking point—where you are really put to the test and challenged by what seems to be an impossible trial—is a lot higher than you might think.

I maintain that getting fit by hiking and climbing is the best thing you can do to ensure that your own personal breaking point is much higher than the norm. It makes you more resilient, more effective at overcoming challenges, more confident, and more self-assured, both at work and in your daily life. Because beyond the physiological benefits, it is also medicine for your spirit and your attitude, for your psyche. The many lessons you will learn will impact both your physical and cognitive health in ways that no other activity can.

## Crucibles

I like to think of some of my outdoor adventures as crucibles. That word isn't used often, but it fits these situations perfectly. The *Oxford Dictionary* defines a crucible as "a situation of severe trial in which different elements interact, leading to the creation of something new." Each time I'm on an outdoor adventure and attempt to go beyond my comfort zone, a new and stronger me is forged.

Nothing you can do in the gym or on the flatlands is the equal of what nature will throw at you in the mountains. It's the unpredictability, the randomness, the unevenness of the terrain that wears at you. Not to mention how the weather (the cold or the heat) and the level of uncertainty add to the degree of difficulty.

One second the ground seems firm; the next second, you may break through the snow cover up to your hips. One minute your ski poles are providing support, the next moment, one of them breaks through the snow crust up to your wrist and pulls you over. A nice, well-marked trail suddenly transitions to a dense forest bushwhack with a bridge-less stream to cross. Add a heavy pack to the situation, and you're constantly fighting for balance and support while moving uphill or downhill. Is that dark shadow a harmless depression or a hidden crevasse? One second you have solid traction, the next second it's wet or icy, and you have to make the necessary adjustments.

Ligaments, tendons, and joints in the feet, ankles, knees, and hips are put to the test over uneven terrain, thousands of times a day. The core muscles of the back and stomach are constantly activated, stressed, and fighting for balance and stability. Lungs are screaming for more air. It can be intense.

That's a crucible. It either breaks you down or, bit by bit, it hardens and strengthens you as nothing else can. And when you develop those mountain legs, you develop a confident, stable mindset, you cannot get elsewhere.

The business world is like that, too—whether it's being an entrepreneur, building something new, owning a small business, pitching customers/partners/investors, or even just going to the office for your daily grind.

You can rewrite your PowerPoint presentation over and over. You can run financial models ad nauseam or build working demos or write memos from the safe space of your desk. But you won't get really good—you won't get your strong workday legs under you—until you get out there and do it and get knocked off balance a few times in the crucible of a competitive marketplace, with real customers, real dollars at stake, and real risk.

The real word has the randomness, the difficulties, and the unpredictability you need to make your plans—and you—stronger, more competitive, and more resilient. That is what makes you more capable of dealing with whatever comes your way.

There's nothing like a crucible—your trial by fire in the real world. And only those who've been through one can truly understand.

## Learn to Love the Uneven Terrain of Life

Recently, I had the pleasure and thrill of trekking across Nepal to Everest Base Camp with legendary mountaineer Peter Hillary, two-time Everest summiteer and lifelong climber and trekker. The occasion was the 100th birthday of Sir Edmund Hillary, his father, who, in 1953 (along with Sherpa Tenzing Norgay), was the first human to stand on the summit of the world's tallest mountain. Peter has crisscrossed Nepal on foot from a very early age, so trekking in with him was a once in a lifetime experience and quite an education in mountain lore.

Of the many parts of this trek that were memorable, Peter's discussions on the concept of "Himalayan flat" stood out more than most. Nepal is the most mountainous country on Earth, the result of the Indian tectonic plate crashing into the Asian plate eons ago, with that collision pushing up the world's tallest mountains. That uplift process created a series of crinkles in the terrain—seemingly never-ending ridges and valleys leading up to the world's highest peaks.

To get to the base of the tallest mountains, one must walk across those ridges and valleys. So, the trek into Everest is far from a smooth, continuous, uphill trek. It's more like 3,000 vertical feet up, 2,000 feet down. Then 4,000 up and 2,000 feet down, followed by 4,000 feet up and 4,000 feet down—repeated for 50 miles.

It's a roller coaster of undulating terrain—so much so, that on some days, you've walked ten rugged miles, gained and lost a lot of altitude, only to finish the day at nearly the same altitude as where you started. You walked all day. Your Fitbit says you've done 20,000 steps and 300 uphill flights, but you end the day no higher than you were in the morning. That's Himalayan Flat. You're exhausted; your body tells you it's been a grueling, long day, but you haven't gained any altitude.

Isn't that exactly what we experience so often in the real world?

## Get Used to the False Summits

Of course, there is also the dreaded false summit to contend with—a particularly challenging illusion that occurs on mountain ridges and is one of the hardest lessons to grasp and digest.

Humans are puny compared to mountains, so there are times as you're walking uphill when you can see a clear point ahead that you believe is the highest point. As you get closer, you come to what you thought was the top, but then suddenly, another higher point appears that was hidden from view. That's a false summit. Sometimes when hiking or climbing a long ridge, you experience a series of false summits. You get close to what you believe is the top and surprise! You see another summit beyond. Then as you approach the top of that one, you see that it's yet another false summit (and sometimes there are several others after that).

One of my favorite hikes in New Hampshire is the Franconia Ridge, a mile-long undulating ridge with three false summits. The first time I did it, even being aware of the false summit phenomenon, I was utterly amazed at how deceptive these false summits could be. I was so sure I was about to come to the high point, only to have my hopes dashed when I saw the next peak, a half-mile away and 500 feet higher. It can rob a person of willpower, demoralize and crush the spirit.

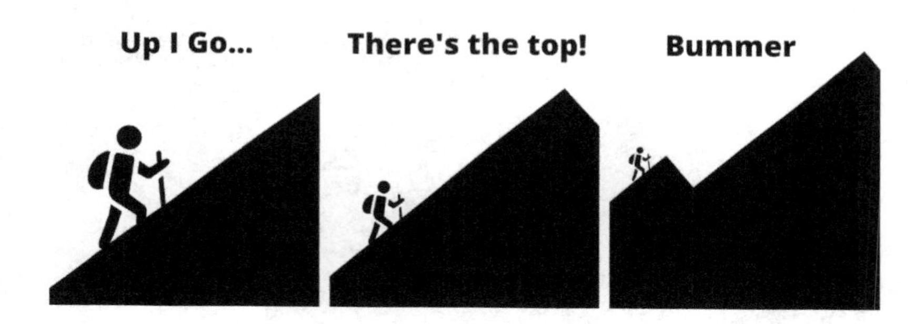


Can you regroup to overcome the obstacle? Over time, you come to the realization that that is just the way it is. There is a very basic principle at work here. In order to get from point A to point B, you cannot fake it. You cannot wish yourself to the top, cannot take a short cut, and can't get someone to carry you. A charming and persuasive personality will not help you here, nor will guile or passing on the responsibility to others. You cannot dodge the problem.

You either move up, or you don't. And when you get up, you have to come down. No excuses.

The purity and directness of this are weighty and scary to some. The effort can strip you down to the core and bring you to tears if you are at your limit. Do you have the willpower, the skill, and the energy to overcome obstacles like the inevitable False Summit?

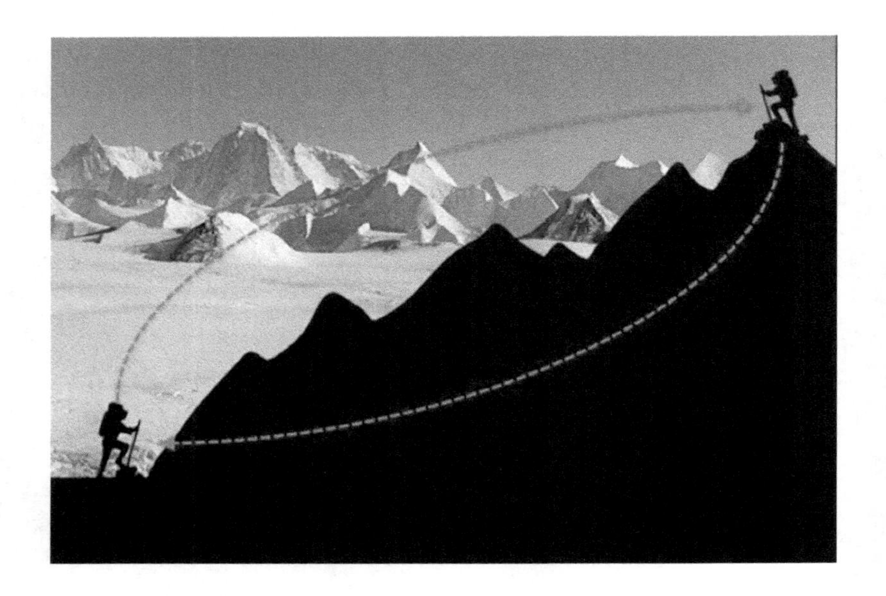

There is no such thing as a simple, easy ride in this life. Few things come easy (perhaps you've heard there is no such thing as a free lunch?). We have ups, and we have downs. Sometimes there are gentle uphills, and other times the going is very rough and steep. Sometimes there's a sharp drop-off, and you are at great risk. Sometimes there are sudden turns that are unpredictable. Sometimes the weather is sunny, and sometimes a sudden storm comes out of nowhere. Sometimes you're following a well-marked trail on a well-made map, and sometimes there is no trail, so you have to make your own path through uncharted territory. Sometimes it's fun, but sometimes it is a long uphill slog, then panic.

What I love most about being outdoors hiking and climbing is that it is the perfect mental preparation for the ups and downs of life. These principles can be applied to business, entrepreneurship, and relationships, and more—anything that causes you to venture outside your comfort zone and into the real world. You learn that ups come with downs, and downs are followed by ups. And you're gaining the tools to navigate whatever comes your way. This is life for anyone who ventures outside their comfort zone into the real world.

## Mental Strength

The physical challenges of exercise have amazing cognitive benefits as well. As Michael Jonesco of Ohio State University explains it:

"The satisfaction of pushing your body and seeing it respond breeds not only a stronger, faster, leaner body, but a more peaceful, satisfied, and confident mind. When you're physically fit, you know firsthand what you can accomplish when you put your mind to it, and you become empowered to hit your personal, career, and relationship goals in a way you wouldn't otherwise" (Fetters 2019).

On a recent trek across Nepal, I had the pleasure of walking with Jenny and Jim Swinden from Melbourne, Australia. Both in their mid-60s, they successfully completed the very demanding 100-mile trek from Lukla to Everest Base Camp and back. They are highly attuned to this aspect of trekking, and Jenny says,

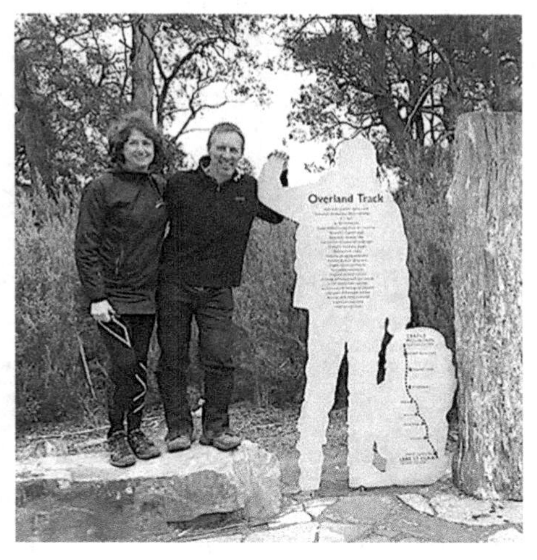


*The Swindons*

"The mental focus that's required to just live in that moment; the only thing you're thinking about is the next few steps. This living-in-the-moment feeling is such a nice change—not to be thinking about things and worried about problems. It's like a meditation in that sense. You're intensely focused on the immediate world. For me, the hook isn't the physical part of this. It's the mental part."

Adds Jim, "When you're on some of these longer walks, you become a different person. You become a trekker. You become a pilgrim; you're living a different lifestyle altogether. You're stepping out of your normal life. You live a lot more simply and learn what you can do without."

These are great lessons to absorb. And truly, most of the time, anything worthwhile in life is not an easy walk up. While you're actually doing it, nothing is ever as easy as it seemed in your dreams. There are usually unexpected setbacks and unplanned obstacles, so you might as well get used to it.

Nature is that kind of teacher, and there is nothing like a mountain to teach that lesson well. Learning to live with reality and losing from time to time is an essential life lesson. Too many people missed that class in school because it's not taught anymore.

## Self-Reliance

In 1993, I joined an expedition to climb the tallest mountain in Antarctica, Mount Vinson. I was eager for this, as I knew something so extreme would be epic and transformative—a crucible. The mountain was so infrequently visited at the time that fewer than 100 people had ever been to the top. When the little Twin Otter plane drops you off at the base of the mountain, you are hundreds of miles away from the nearest human beings. And of course, there is no cell signal.

Standing alone atop a remote wilderness peak, especially in extreme conditions, you can fully appreciate and completely assimilate the importance of the skill of self-reliance, and that was exactly the crucible I needed at the time.

So, to intensify the sense of being alone and self-reliant, on a rest day about halfway up the mountain, I decided to make a solo, side trip to a small, neighboring sub-peak. My three companions and I were alone, hundreds of miles from the nearest humans, but I wanted to be more isolated still, to see what that was like.

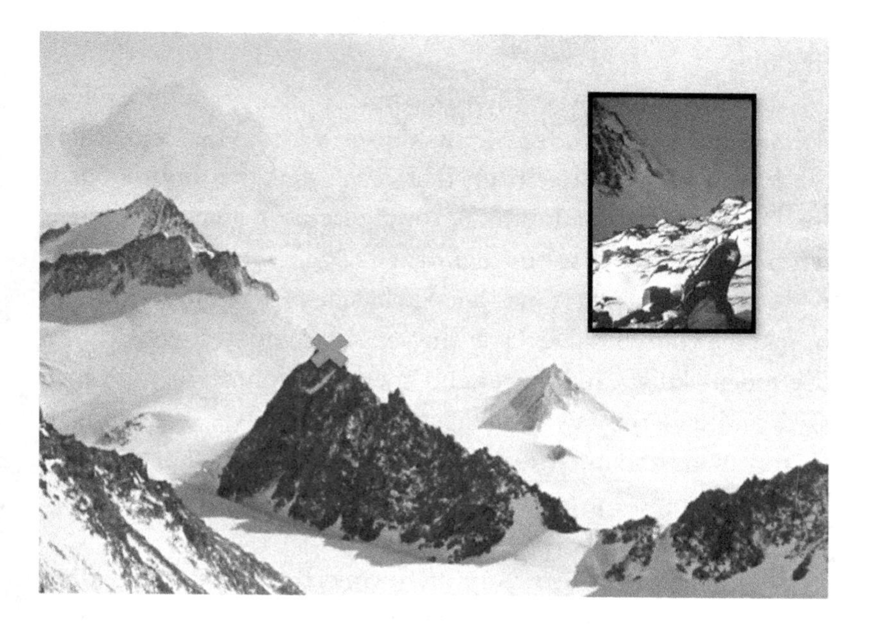

I climbed two miles across a glacier, up a rocky, narrow ridge to the red X in the photo. It was ten degrees below zero. I sat down with my foot hanging over the edge on a pinnacle, where one misstep would be fatal, and no other human being on earth knew where I was or would ever find me if something went badly wrong. The conditions in this spot are cold enough to freeze boiling water instantly. The snow squeaks like Styrofoam and exposed skin will be frostbitten very quickly. And it was two steep miles back down to the relative safety and warmth of the tent and my three companions. I sat there and soaked it all in for an hour, knowing I was probably the first person to ever be in that spot. I still find it amazing that a single hour—almost 30 years ago—is still with me every single day.

You instantly develop a heightened sense of absolute self-reliance in such situations, because without it, just staying alive for a month until the plane returns can be difficult in a place like that.

The rest of the expedition was fine (amazing really), and we summited and descended Mount Vinson without incident. There are lots of other stories from that climb, but that hour I spent totally alone, exposed, and beyond rescue if something went wrong, remains, by far, the highlight.

Of course, hanging over a ledge in sub-zero weather does not have to be your crucible. Over the years, step by step, you acquire the tools, skills, experience, and mental fortitude to minimize risks and take on new challenges with confidence. You learn to trust yourself and not just survive, but to thrive. Truly, at the time, I was so competent and confident in myself, that I was not the least bit concerned for my safety.

So here it is, in short: Your life shrinks or expands depending on your level of willingness to accept risk and to stretch the limits of your comfort zone. Your life expands exponentially if you seek the transformative power of a crucible.

# 19

# ALWAYS SEEKING ANOTHER SUMMIT

*When you get to the top of the mountain, keep climbing.*

— ZEN PARABLE

That is exactly what I intend to do. Each hill, each summit, is merely a stepping-stone to the next. I am addicted—not to standing on summits, but to the effort of heading uphill. The purity of one foot in front of the other, the strain it puts on muscles and lungs, is not hard work for me. It is pleasure. The feeling of accomplishment from moving uphill, no matter how high that hill may be, is a reward in itself. The joy of standing on a summit, a ridge walk, or an open vista, with wind in the trees or the rush of a mountain stream or overlooking a pristine snowfield or fall colors—all these are wonderful bonuses. There are no bad days in the mountains for me.

So, I'll say it one final time: You can do this too. Just take the first few little steps. If you are at all apprehensive, simply step outside your comfort zone just a tiny bit. It's infectious and addictive. It stretches you, and it adds up over time to big gains.

You will never know what you are capable of unless you get out there. Hiking is not only the closest thing we have to The Fountain of Youth, but it is also free medicine—upstream preventive healthcare that can completely change the trajectory of the way we age. It creates a life force that can transform and invigorate every aspect of your life.

These are nice sentiments and easy words to say. But do more than that. Turn these words into action. Do it. Take the first steps. Walk, train, get outside, hike, and experience this for yourself.

If you push it too far at first and exceed your current abilities, simply back off, train a bit harder, and either try again or find another, smaller goal. I do this on an on-going basis, and I always have. I make plans—I think big, look beyond my comfort zone, try things out,

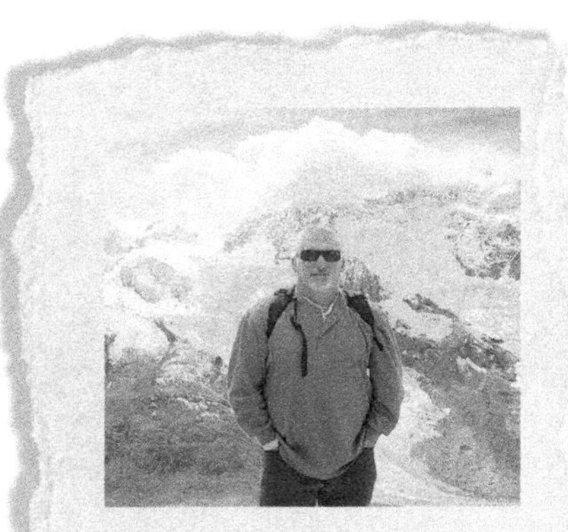

*Hiking beneath Liskamm, Switzerland*

I love going back to the sites of epic adventures from years ago and seeing the summits from a distance, from far below. That's Liskamm, a 14,852-foot peak near Zermatt in the Swiss Alps. 20 years ago!

"You cannot stay on the summit forever. You have to come down again. So, what's the point? Only this: what is above knows what is below, what is below does not know what is above ...

"There is an art to finding your way in the lower regions by the memory of what you have seen when you were higher up. When you can no longer see, you can at least still know."

– Mount Analogue, Rene Daumal

test myself in a crucible, and adjust those plans as needed if I go too far. (Like planning to climb the tallest mountain in the world in my 60s.)

## My Everest Crucible

I went to Mount Everest in Nepal last year, because climbing it has been on my to-do list for decades. Every serious mountaineer aspires to stand on top of the tallest mountain on the planet, 29,028 feet above sea level. It's the height that planes fly, where the oxygen level is 32 percent of normal, and the temperature, on a good day, can be -30° F (or lower).

Up there is called "the death zone" for a good reason. Lack of oxygen makes you colder, it makes your muscles weaker, and it reduces your endurance. Hair, beard, and fingernails stop growing. It's hard to digest food. It kills brain cells. It's dangerous. So, the idea is to get up and down the mountain as quickly as possible—out of danger and back down to the lower altitudes. To do that, you need to be supremely fit, very experienced, and also very lucky.

Sure, it seems senseless and risky to most, but not to a lifelong mountaineer. With the many peaks I've summited, it was the obvious missing jewel in my collection. I can count more than a dozen people I've climbed with over the years who have been atop Everest multiple times and returned safely. So, it has never seemed so outlandish to me, despite the death zone and the sensationalized, annual fatalities.

But at age 63, I did not delude myself that reaching the summit would be easy. I was not the same climber I was at 35, and though very fit, there are certain undeniable physiological factors that age brings to the equation. It increases the risk and the possibility that being at that extreme altitude would be extra challenging. I also climb a bit slower now, potentially increasing the time spent in the death zone.

Still, this wasn't a naively unrealistic goal. The mountain has been climbed by 80-year-old Yuichiro Miura (after recovering from heart surgery!). And though rare, others in their 60s and 70s have summited. Even so, being quite cautious for a risk-taker, I needed to give my goal a reality test before fully committing to the summit attempt.

The plan was to trek into Base Camp, get to 18,000 feet above sea level, and scope it out, up close. If all went well, and my body easily acclimated, I'd boost my training intensity when I got home, climb a few minor peaks in Nepal the next year, and then head back to Everest for a summit attempt.

So then, off I went to Kathmandu and to Everest.

It was a truly marvelous trek. I joined a group of friends that included two Everest summiteers, my old friend Robert Mads Andersen and my new friend Peter Hillary. The occasion was the 100th birthday of Sir Edmund Hillary, Peter's father. And so, this trek was called "In the Footsteps of Hillary," and was it ever.

Every step of the way over the three-week, 100-mile journey was on the same route trodden by Sir Edmund and the 1953 British Everest Expedition, the first to succeed. It was magnificent, drenched in the history of the region and the colorful villages and monasteries along the way, and decorated by the surreal vistas of the world's tallest mountains. Every evening, we talked about the legends of these hills—stories absorbed by both Peter and Robert after lifetimes of adventures here.

These discussions were not only mesmerizing, but they also distracted me from a growing concern: the higher we got, even allowing for proper acclimatization to the higher altitudes, the worse my sleep became, both in duration and in quality. At about 15,000 feet above sea level, where the oxygen levels are only 58 percent of normal, I developed the dreaded Cheyne-Stokes breathing. This is an irregular breathing pattern related to sleep apnea and is not uncommon at high altitude.

I was fine when moving and trekking during the day. But trying to fall asleep triggered it. Gasping for air, I had sensations of drowning and claustrophobia. The higher we got, the worse my nighttime breathing got. This condition will often improve over time with better acclimatization, but no such luck for me.

My sleep plummeted down to just a few fitful hours per night, which is just not enough for muscles or the brain to fully recover from the exertion of high-altitude trekking, and higher up on the mountain, it can have fatal consequences. It also has the effect of weakening the body's defenses and immune system, so you become susceptible to infections, and your system uses extra resources trying to protect you, which then causes additional fatigue.

After three or four days of that, the coughing started, also a fairly common occurrence at altitude, before you are fully acclimated, but in this case, I'd picked up a germ somewhere along the way (again, not uncommon here) and that turned into a serious lung infection—at Everest Base Camp, of all places.

More than halfway up Everest is not exactly a convenient place to get sick, much less in the lungs, when the oxygen level is already diminished by almost 50 percent. So my choices became, a) remain there and hope for recovery and better acclimatization; b) call for an expensive helicopter rescue to get back to lower altitudes that same day; or c) walk out—over 50 miles and five days of undulating Himalayan Flats, back to the airstrip, where I could fly back to Kathmandu.

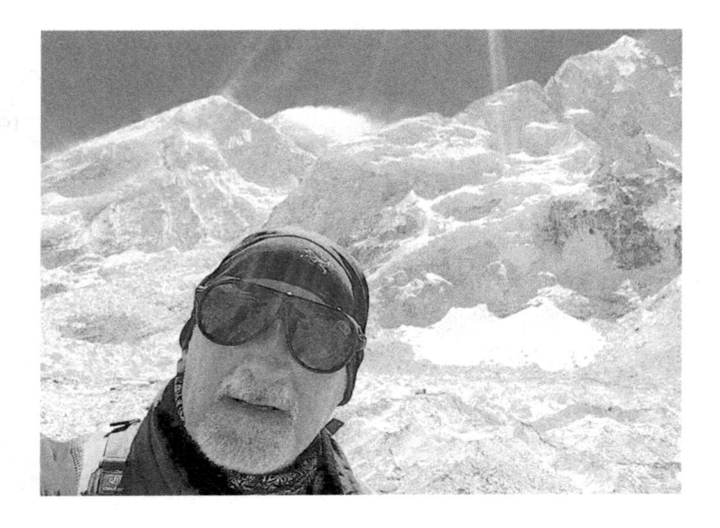

*At Everest Base Camp*

Option a was not possible; we were on a schedule. I opted for the walk-out, hoping that the massive antibiotics I was now taking would stem the infection and permit me to descend under my own power. So, along with my Sherpa friend Balbahadur Shrestha, we left the group a few days early and headed down, hoping that we made the right decision.

We did.

It was by no means easy. It was like trying to do a strenuous hike when weakened by a bad case of the flu. The undulating terrain, though mostly downhill, had enough steep uphill to make those sections a bit of a struggle, even with Bal's assist of carrying much of my gear. I lost my voice as well and may have coughed up part of a lung, but with each day, the breathing got a little easier. The Cheyne Stokes breathing vanished, and blissful, restorative, brain-cleansing sleep returned at about 11,000 feet above sea level, in Namche Bazaar.

Back safely in Kathmandu, it was time to re-assess my plan to return the next year and try for the summit. I had gone to Everest well aware that the ability to tolerate altitude changes with age and assumed that I could overcome that with a combination of extra training and years of experience. Instead, I learned I probably should not return the next year for a summit attempt. I might not be able to acclimate to the altitude. There is probably too much risk. It may now be beyond me.

But guess what? I'm ok with that.

Not achieving an Everest summit will not stop me from heading uphill as often as I can to receive the brain and body benefits of the mountains. Climbing it was, admittedly, a long shot. I should have crossed it off the list 25 years ago. And I don't want it so badly that I'm going to be stupid about it. It's an amazingly big world, with many other hills, many other challenging tests to stretch my comfort zone, and an infinite number of ways to receive all the benefits of outside, uphill, hiking—to find awe and joy, without taking the extreme risk of trying to summit Everest at age 64.

Instead, I have a new to-do list for the next few years:

1. A return pilgrimage to Japan to climb Mount Fuji with some pals from high school
2. Finishing the New Hampshire 48—all forty-eight 4,000-foot peaks in the State (I'm at 35 now)
3. The 270+ mile Long Trail in Vermont (if I can manage three weeks off!)
3. A few of the 14ers (the 14,000+ foot mountains) in Colorado
4. Mount Whitney, the tallest peak in California (in winter)
5. Something in Nepal within view of Everest (it's addictive)

6. The Haute Route, or parts of it, in the French-Swiss Alps
7. Running up the Empire State Building for charity.

What are you planning for the next few years?

It's not important what, specifically, is on the list. What is most important is actually having the list. Who knows if I will get all of this done. Something else will likely be added, and something will fall off the list. The important thing is this: **Always make plans.**

Aging is relentless. You have to stay ahead of it, or it catches up with you. So, having something to look forward to, having the optimism and positive attitude to make far-off, future plans is essential. It's one of the keys to longevity.

Hiking helps you to think in this way because the more you do it, the more blood and oxygen you are pumping through your brain. The mental high you get from this keeps you thinking positively, keeps you optimistic, and purges you of stress and anger, gives you additional perspective on things, and that naturally leads to making plans for the next hike. And that spills over into everything you do.

Perhaps you've heard health and wellness guru Dr. Michael Mantell's life rules, "Rule #1: Don't sweat the small stuff. Rule #2: It's all small stuff." The mountains will help you see the truth in those statements. They have certainly given me that perspective. When I forget this, my solution is to go for a hike, and then everything else falls into place. Any lingering doubts fade. Calmness and focus are restored, and optimism and enthusiasm return.

In fact, this works so well, that with the hindsight of a year to think about it, I'm wondering what would happen if I went back to Everest, better trained, and without a lung infection? Could I? We shall see.

There are never any guarantees about what's ahead or promises about living a long life. There are too many variables. So, I'm just going to keep planning and keep walking uphill, one foot in front of the other, until I can't do it anymore.

I'm always seeking another trail, another hill, another vista, another summit. I'm on a never-ending adventure. I'm heading up trails with no idea what's around the bend, or past the next false summit. But I can't wait to find out.

## *The End*

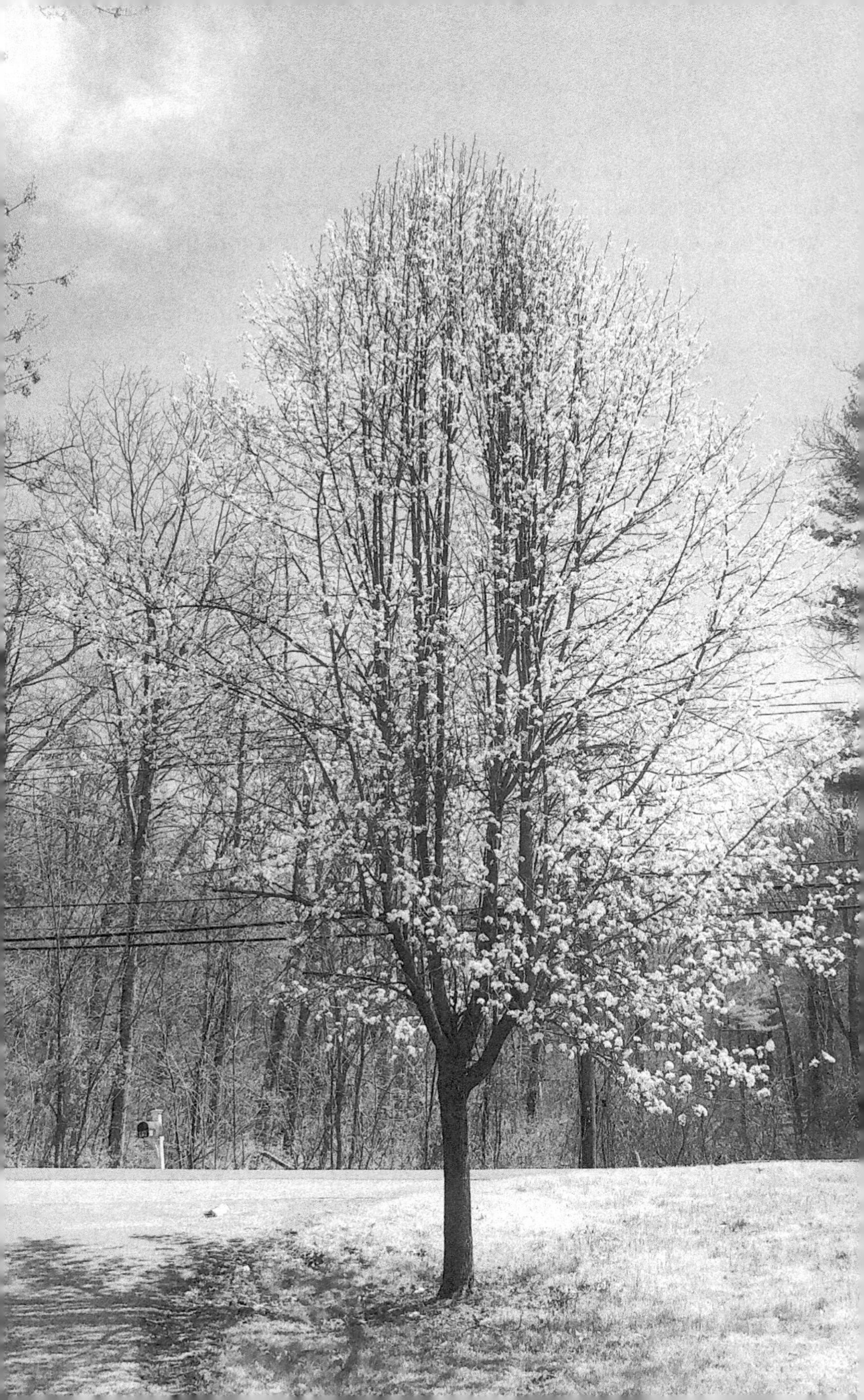

# EPILOGUE

*I have seen many storms in my life. Most storms have caught me by surprise, so I had to learn very quickly to look further and understand that I am not capable of controlling the weather, to exercise the art of patience and to respect the fury of nature.*

— PAULO COELHO

This Bradford Pear tree was my birthday present about 25 years ago. During a freak October snowstorm about 10 years ago, the top of it snapped off. Early snow, when all the leaves are still on the trees, has a tendency to create overload from the extreme weight it creates. All that was left was the trunk and a few small branches.

The sensible thing would have been to cut it down. But there were so many other fallen trees and branches downed after that storm, we never got around to this one. Maybe I didn't have the heart to remove it when the time came. It was "my tree," and I wanted to wait until spring to see what would happen.

Well, in March, the tree began to flower and grow. Although it looked badly broken and disfigured, I still could not bear to give up on it. Tree experts said it would never survive, and I almost cut it down several times. A lot of people thought it was not worthy of its position at the end of the driveway.

But, little by little, it came back to life. And each year, new vertical branches sprouted and multiplied where there had been just one main trunk.

Cut to the present. My tree is a totally unique, one-of-a-kind, magnificent Bradford Pear with seven strong vertical branches that magnify its mid-April to late-May flowering beauty. It always reminds me of the spirit of spring—the annual fresh start and reawakening of what had been dormant. In full bloom, it is a big, glowing ball of white flowers.

Well, its leaves popped a couple of days ago, right in the middle of the coronavirus pandemic. Now, more than ever, it reminds me that there is great hope in patience, perseverance, and the natural ability to heal and then thrive again.

The moral of this story? No matter how low things seem to be, or how down you are, don't give up on something damaged or seemingly beyond repair. Nature shows us that patience, perseverance, and an optimistic vision of a brighter future can prevail. As I write this in spring 2020, we're all feeling a bit battered and unsure, but with perseverance, we will also recover and thrive.

Be well,

*Martin Pazzani*

*Secrets of Aging Well: Get Outside*

GetOutside.online
martin@GetOutside.online
April 26, 2020

# ABOUT THE AUTHOR

Martin Pazzani is a global business executive, a fitness entrepreneur, and an avid hiker, trekker, and mountaineer. Over 50 years, he has taken 100,000,000 uphill steps across seven continents.

Throughout his long business career, he's worn many hats—strategist, chief marketing officer, CEO, company founder, advertising guy, management consultant, speaker, and burger flipper. The companies have ranged from tiny startups to international mega-corporations. Over an equally long period of time, he's pursued peaks from Antarctica to Nepal and across Europe, Africa, and North and South America.

At age 64, he's not slowing down one bit and currently juggles three start-ups in fitness, craft spirits, and marketing communications. He stays active and youthful through hiking, trekking, and climbing. His brain fitness think tank, Act!vate Brain & Body, is focused on the health and longevity of active agers and they are on a mission to radically improve the trajectory of aging.

Martin has given seminars, talks, and keynote speeches to thousands of Fortune 1000 executives, colleagues, and clients at corporate headquarters, retreats, and venues as varied as the Cannes Lions Ad Festival, The TED Conference in Monterrey, California, the Dubai Lynx Show, The Copacabana Palace in Rio de Janeiro, and New York's Waldorf Astoria Hotel. His talks can teach, motivate, and inspire with a combination of gravitas, expertise, and joy.

Find more at **GetOutside.online** and **MartinPazzani.com**.
Book him to speak to your group at
**martin@GetOutside.online**

---

*"I am always learning."*

– **Michelangelo Buonarroti** at age 87

---

# WORKS CITED


American Cancer Society. 2016. "Exercise Linked With Lower Risk of 13 Types of Cancer." May 17. https://www.cancer.org/latest-news/exercise-linked-with-lower-risk-of-13-types-of-cancer.html.

Arvesen, Amelia. 2019. *snews*. September 20. https://www.snewsnet.com/news/outdoor-recreation-427-billion?fbclid=IwAR0b9P1Y_khp0ym7Hn8z7o-x-bB5pqTgExYyBJ3JJGEp9Y4l1_Kmh-OkmvA.

Averill, Graham. 2020. *Outside Online*. January 16. https://www.outsideonline.com/2407738/100-year-old-klaus-obermeyer-skier.

Ballantyne, Coco. 2009. "Does Exercise Really Make You Healthier?" January 2. https://www.scientificamerican.com/article/does-exercise-really-make/.

Carter, Kenneth. 2020. "Lust for Life." *Psychology Today*, October 15: 78-88.

Center For Disease Control and Prevention. 2020. *National Center for Health Statistics*. https://www.cdc.gov/nchs/fastats/leading-causes-of-death.htm.

Cheng, Michelle & Kopf, Dan. 2019. "The Number of Americans Working in Their 70s is Skyrocketing." June 3. https://qz.com/work/1632602/the-number-of-americans-working-in-their-70s-is-skyrocketing/.

Cleveland Clinic Newsroom. 2019. "Can Obesity Impact the Size of Your Brain?" March 2019. https://newsroom.clevelandclinic.org/2019/03/12/can-obesity-impact-the-size-of-your-brain/.

Crouch, Michelle. 2019. "To Live Longer, Exercise Daily." January 8. https://www.aarp.org/health/healthy-living/info-2019/exercise-longevity-wellness-benefits.html.

Design Fitness Center. 2019. *Design Fitness Center*. March 10. https://www.designfitnesscentre.com/healthfitness-blog/studies-link-obesity-to-smaller-brains.

2019. *Diabetes and Obesity*. January 15. https://www.diabetes.co.uk/diabetes-and-obesity.html.

Fetters, K. Aleisha. 2019. *Everyday Health*. May 22. https://www.everydayhealth.com/everything-you-need-know-about-fitness-why-its-about-way-more-than-hitting-gym/.

Fowler, Danielle. 2019. May 17. https://finance.yahoo.com/news/fast-walkers-longer-life-expectancy-120210928.html?ncid=facebook_yfsocialfa_wje3x23a50w&utm_content=bufferbf522&utm_medium=social&utm_source=facebook.com&utm_campaign=yahoofinance&fbclid=IwAR3XKpz5pO86Ke1_VA_sXe-S58DO3VToUMumQ64TsEdfSNfhYizntTRb6X4.

Futurity. 2016. *Futurity*. January 12. http://www.futurity.org/obesity-sedentary-behavior-1089352-2/.

Greville, Georgia. 2017. *The Outbound Collective*. May 4. Accessed May 4, 2017. https://www.theoutbound.com/georgiagreville/12-reasons-why-you-should-spend-more-time-outdoors?fbclid=IwAR0nZdSn4CX9z9sf_lMMQzACUG09PrR5UTTE84M4Khf42ur_fz-BW01RfuI.

Haynes, Trevor. 2020. *Harvard.edu*. http://sitn.hms.harvard.edu/flash/2018/dopamine-smartphones-battle-time/.

Heid, Markham. 2017. *Time.com*. July 5. https://time.com/4820394/hiking-walking-mind-body-workout/?fbclid=IwAR2zwYNXnZeA_ULdph14NyUd_kYeSfaZD5Gh3kTcAJiv3KSbv29I3QRs06M.

Jeurissen, Al. 2003. "The effects of physical exercise on the immune system." *PubMed.gov*, July 12.

LaPonsie, Maryalene. 2018. "Could an Early Retirement Help You Live Longer?" June 21. https://money.usnews.com/money/retirement/articles/2018-06-21/could-an-early-retirement-help-you-live-longer.

Lemar, Marissa Cruz. 2019. "Never Exercised in Your Life? It's Not Too Late to Start — and Benefit." October 21. https://www.washingtonpost.com/lifestyle/wellness/never-exercised-in-your-life-its-not-too-late-to-start--and-benefit/2019/10/18/fd9b9342-f037-11e9-b648-76bcf86eb67e_story.html?fbclid=IwAR3-YLwRFE8BbU0m9LqxIE9A-syrCncECMz5tB4UN5lgSRy1o6zpfi23zMg.

Martin, Stephen. 2009. "NCBI." *NCBI*. October 1. https://www.ncbi.nlm.nih.gov/pmc/articles/PMC2803113/.

Mayo Clinic. 2014. "Slowing or Reversing Muscle Loss." April 10. https://www.mayoclinic.org/medical-professionals/physical-medicine-rehabilitation/news/slowing-or-reversing-muscle-loss/mac-20431104.

—. 2019. "Your secret weapon during cancer treatment? Exercise!" June 11. https://www.mayoclinic.org/diseases-conditions/cancer/in-depth/secret-weapon-during-cancer-treatment-exercise/art-20457584.

Medical News Today. 2019. *Medical News Today*. August 6. https://www.medicalnewstoday.com/articles/.

Merchant, Nilofer. 2014. *Harvard Business Review*. August 7. https://hbr.org/2013/01/sitting-is-the-smoking-of-our-generation.

—. 2014. *Harvard Business Review*. August 7. https://hbr.org/2013/01/sitting-is-the-smoking-of-our-generation.

2020. "Mindfulness." *Psychology Today*.

Mohonk Mountain House. 2020. Mohonk Mountain House. Accessed 2020. https://www.mohonk.com/spa/mindfulness/?gclid=CjwKCAiA35rxBRAWEiwADqB37-ATJNfJdiUrCK3mXo1pPeAk9DhHGYFh-uPbQIStVlUxjxWoqjHcIRoCDooQAvD_BwE.

NICM, Western Sydney University. 2017. "Exercise Increases Brain Size, New Research Finds." November 13. https://www.sciencedaily.com/releases/2017/11/171113195024.htm.

O'BRIEN, CHRIS. February. *L.A. Times*. 26 2013. Accessed 26 2013, February. https://www.latimes.com/business/la-xpm-2013-feb-26-la-fi-tn-ted-2013-nilofer-merchant-says-sitting-is-the-new-smoking-20130226-story.html.

2014. "Piper Jaffray Fitness Industry Report."

Psychology Today. 2020. *Psychology Today*. January 1. Accessed January 1, 2020. https://www.psychologytoday.com/us/basics/mindfulness.

Schondelmeyer, Stephen W. and Purvis, Leigh. September . *AARP*. 2018 1. Accessed 2018 1, September . https://www.aarp.org/content/dam/aarp/ppi/2018/09/trends-in-retail-prices-of-brand-name-prescription-drugs-year-end-update.pdf.

Schultheis, Rob. 1986. *One Man's Search for the Ultimate Athletic High*. International Publishing.

Sherry Christiansen. 2018. *Alzheimers.net*. August 13. https://www.alzheimers.net/the-cost-of-dementia-care/.

Sifferlin, Alexandra. 2018. *Time.com*. February 20. https://time.com/5166564/physical-exercise-can-increase-lifespan/.

Society for Neuroscience. 2020. "A New Role For Neurogenesis." January 20. https://medicalxpress.com/news/2020-01-role-neurogenesis.html.

Stephen Schondelmeyer, Leigh Purvis. 2018. *AARP*. September. https://www.aarp.org/content/dam/aarp/ppi/2018/09/trends-in-retail-prices-of-brand-name-prescription-drugs-year-end-update.pdf.

University of East Anglia. 2018. "It's Official - Spending Time Outside is Good for You." June 7. https://www.uea.ac.uk/about/-/it-s-official-spending-time-outside-is-good-for-you.

White, Mathew. 2019. Science News. June 19. Accessed June 19, 2019. https://www.sciencedaily.com/releases/2019/06/190613095227.htm?fbclid=IwAR0p7WtGqwt8u0m_8PhG2ekKj7dOnqW1tWKuWLjzbfFYEryGEix-DD48f28.

Wikipedia. 2020. *Wikipedia*. Accessed 2020. https://en.wikipedia.org/wiki/Mindfulness.

Wittkowsk, Professor Knut. 2020. *YouTube*. April 3. https://www.youtube.com/watch?v=lGC5sGdz4kg&fbclid=IwAR1SkwkoUCvBguRJidX-eMB6O0s7G6FuECP1kHsAHlr2_vTX4rvvbPGUS08.

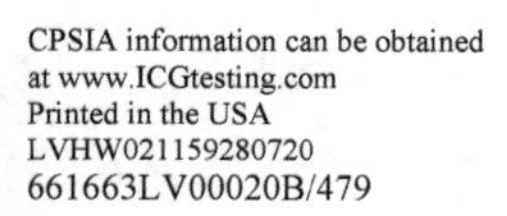

CPSIA information can be obtained
at www.ICGtesting.com
Printed in the USA
LVHW021159280720
661663LV00020B/479